D0147235

HEALTH SCIENCES LIBRARY
WITHDRAWN HOSPITAL
3024 Fairfield Avenue
Fort Wayne, Indiana 46807-1697

Dying and Disabled Children: Dealing with Loss and Grief

Dying and Disabled Children: Dealing with Loss and Grief

Harold M. Dick, David Price Roye, Jr.,
Penelope R. Buschman, Austin H. Kutscher,
Boris Rubinstein, and Francis K. Forstenzer
Editors

The Haworth Press
New York • London

Dying and Disabled Children: Dealing with Loss and Grief has also been published as *Loss, Grief & Care*, Volume 2, Numbers 3/4 1988.

© 1988 by The Haworth Press, Inc. All rights reserved. No part of this book may be reproduced or utilized in any form or by any means, electronic or mechanical, including photocopying, microfilm and recording, or by any information storage and retrieval system, without permission in writing from the publisher. Printed in the United States of America.

The Haworth Press, Inc., 12 West 32 Street, New York, NY 10001
EUROSPAN/Haworth, 3 Henrietta Street, London WC2E 8LU England

LIBRARY OF CONGRESS
Library of Congress Cataloging-in-Publication Data

Dying and disabled children: dealing with loss and grief / Harold M.
    Dick ... [et al.], editors.
      p. cm.
    "Has also been published as Loss, grief & care, volume 2, numbers
3/4, 1988" – T.p. verso.
    Includes bibliographies.
    ISBN 0-86656-759-3
    1. Physically handicapped children – Psychology. 2. Terminally ill children – Psychology.
3. Sick children – Family relationships. 4. Children and death. I. Dick, Harold M.
RJ47.5.D95 1988
155.9'37 – dc 19   88-15364
                                          CIP

Dying and Disabled Children: Dealing with Loss and Grief

CONTENTS

ABOUT THE EDITORS

Harold M. Dick, MD, is Director of Orthopedic Surgery Service at the Presbyterian Hospital, Columbia-Presbyterian Medical Center. He is also Frank E. Stinchfield Professor and Chairman of the Department of Orthopedic Surgery at the College of Physicians and Surgeons, Columbia University, in New York City. As a specialist in orthopedic surgery, especially hand surgery, Dr. Dick provides consultation to many hospitals.

David Price Roye, Jr., MD, is Chief of Pediatric Orthopedics at Babies Hospital, Columbia-Presbyterian Medical Center. He is also Assistant Professor of Clinical Orthopedic Surgery at the College of Physicians and Surgeons, Columbia University, in New York City. Dr. Roye has lectured nationwide and published many articles in the area of pediatric orthopedics.

Penelope R. Buschman, RN, MS, is Assistant Professor of Clinical Nursing at Columbia University School of Nursing. She is also Research Nurse Clinician at the Presbyterian Hospital in New York City, where she provides care to chronically and terminally ill children and families and consultation to the nursing and medical staff.

Austin H. Kutscher is President of The Foundation of Thanatology and Professor of Dentistry (in Psychiatry) at the College of Physicians and Surgeons, Columbia University, in New York City. His clinical and teaching activities have focused on psychosocial aspects of life-threatening illness and bereavement; cancer diagnosis, therapy and management; and pharmacotherapeutics. Dr. Kutscher is the editor of *Loss, Grief & Care*.

Boris Rubinstein, MD, MPH, is Director of The Pediatric Psychiatry Consultation and Liaison Service at Babies Hospital, Columbia-Presbyterian Medical Center in New York City. At Babies Hospital, he is a consultant to orthopedists, surgeons, and pediatricians on the psychological factors that affect physical illness. Dr. Rubinstein is also a child psychiatrist in private practice in Westchester, New York. He has written previously on the psychiatric aspects of chronic handicaps.

Frances K. Forstenzer, LCSW, is Intake and Family Services Coordinator for Return, a program for head-injured adults at Sinai Hospital of Baltimore, Maryland. She is also a field work supervisor for the University of Maryland School of Social Work and Community Planning, and has a private psychotherapy practice in Baltimore. Her previous publications include an article on support groups for the parents of physically handicapped children.

Dying and Disabled Children: Dealing with Loss and Grief

I. LOSS OF A BODY PART

Traumatic Amputation in Childhood: Functional and Psychosocial Aspects

John R. Denton

Amputation is a surgical procedure that has a sense of finality. This is perceived by both the operating surgeon and the patient. The amputated part is gone forever. The amputation stump may be revised, but it can never be converted. This sense of permanent loss separates amputations from all other surgical procedures.

Amputation surgery is one of the oldest modalities of our discipline. The first amputation followed by the fitting of a prosthesis was recorded around 3,000 B.C. (VanDerwerker 1976). A warrior queen lost her leg in battle and was fitted with an iron leg with which she could lead her people back into conflict. In 500 B.C., Hippocrates wrote a treatise, "On Joints," in which he recommended amputation as the treatment for gangrene. An Italian vase, circa 400 B.C., depicts for the first time a patient using a pylon prosthesis. The European wars produced increasing numbers of amputees as a result of the continued sophistication of gunnery, coupled with the clumsiness of outdated battlefield tactics. Then, in the

John R. Denton, MD, is Chief, Pediatric Orthopedic Service, Columbia-Presbyterian Medical Center. He is also Associate Professor of Orthopedic Surgery, College of Physicians and Surgeons, Columbia University, New York, NY.

© 1988 by The Haworth Press, Inc. All rights reserved.

second half of the nineteenth century, two medical events occurred that placed amputation surgery on a more modern path. These two landmark events, the recognition of the principle of asepsis and the discovery of general anesthesia, not only made it possible to treat some wounds without amputation, but allowed the stumps of amputated limbs to be fashioned into more serviceable condition. The advent of antibiotics, just prior to World War II, followed in the 1940s and 50s by advances in vascular surgery, forever changed statistics on amputations as a consequence of wounding.

Despite these advances, there are still indications for traumatic amputations. The classic indication is an irreparable loss of blood supply to a part; a second indication is such extensive damage to the bone and soft tissue of the part that healing is not possible; the third indication is an injury of such magnitude that when surgeons contemplate the long healing time involved, the need for prolonged hospitalizations and surgeries, still coupled with an uncertain result, they conclude that amputation will provide a limb that will be just as serviceable. A relative indication is the development of infection, usually gas gangrene, a few days after a limb has been injured, so that if the limb is not amputated, the infection threatens the life of the patient. Over the past ten years, the advancement of microsurgery and replantation surgery, as well as the use of external fixators for severely traumatized limbs, have been valuable additions to the armamentarium available to surgeons in the effort to salvage badly injured limbs.

Amputations in childhood are of two types: (1) congenital, by which we include later ablation of a deformed limb or part of a limb, and (2) acquired, which includes the two classic categories of traumatic and elective, such as for tumor or other disease. When amputations are necessary because of a tumor, infection, or limb deformity, they are planned and prepared for by the patients and their families. In these cases, the part that is to be amputated is not "normal" and, indeed, may be a threat to the child's life. The affected limb is often a source of pain or is a functional handicap; this type of amputation can be seen as getting rid of an abnormal limb that is causing problems. In contrast, the traumatic amputation differs from others in that it is not prepared for by patients or their families. For example, when a normal, healthy child leaves for school at 7:30 AM and later the family receives a telephone call from the emergency room informing them that the child has been in an accident and has lost a limb, there has been no time for emotional preparation. When a healthy child loses a normal limb, the sudden emotional shock to both the parents and the child cannot be overstated. In this article, both the functional and psychosocial aspects of this kind of calamity will be addressed.

Currently, the most common causes of childhood amputations are (1) explosives (which usually cause amputations of an upper extremity), (2) motor vehicle accidents, (3) power tools, including power mowers and snowblowers, (4) railroad accidents, and (5) thermal injuries. An excellent, up-to-date publication in this field is the *Journal of the Association of Children's Prosthetic-Orthotic Clinics*, published by Ms. Joan Edelstein at New York University (Edelstein 1985). This new publication is an outgrowth of the familiar *Inter-Clinic Informational Bulletin*, which contains state-of-the-art articles on both prosthetic and orthotic devices as well as the psychosocial dimensions of the problem. It is a reference that should be in every child amputee clinic.

FUNCTIONAL ASPECTS

In general, children do extremely well with amputations. The well-known axiom that children are not small adults and are different from adults could be modified to state that child amputees are *very* different from adult amputees. Data indicate that almost 100 percent of lower extremity child amputees use a prosthesis; 75 percent of upper extremity child amputees use a prosthesis at least part of the time (Suderman, Tervo, and Leszczynski 1982). These figures are vastly different from those of older dysvascular amputees. For the most part, child amputees do not have the other systemic problems that limit older amputees. To amplify the benefit of youth, it is noted that the younger the child amputee, the quicker and more facile he or she becomes at using a prosthesis. Children more quickly incorporate the prosthesis into their body image. Children are not reluctant to demonstrate the use of their prosthesis or to discuss it.

The level of amputation in children should be a disarticulation, if possible (Tooms 1980). This accomplishes two purposes: (1) it maintains a growth plate and (2) it diminishes the occurrence of ectopic bone and spurring at the tip of the stump. The first point is extremely important, particularly in younger children. For example, a child who sustains a mid-thigh amputation at age four will have a very short stump at age sixteen, since growth will occur only from the proximal femoral growth plate, which grows only at the rate of 0.3 centimeters annually. In the same child, a knee disarticulation, which preserves the distal femoral growth plate, would grow an additional 9.0 centimeters in length, since this growth plate has a yearly growth of 0.9 centimeters. In the latter case, the child will have an adequate length stump for prosthetic fitting. If, when the patient reached maturity, the stump was too long, a revision could be done.

When possible, an immediate fit rigid dressing should be applied in the operating room. Although dressing might be done at the stage of delayed primary closure rather than at the primary amputation, the immediate fit rigid dressing provides better wound healing: the patient "awakens with the leg"; the patient begins ambulation earlier; and there is better control of edema. The only contraindications to this rigid dressing are a contaminated wound that involves frequent wound inspection or an amputation that is left open for secondary closure later.

Another difference between child and adult amputees is the growth, both in girth and length, of the child's stump. This necessitates appropriate adjustments by the prosthetist and the purchase of a new limb every two to four years. Also, because children are good prosthetic users and are very active, they have a higher rate of breakage and repair of their prostheses. This is actually a "good problem" to have, since it indicates that the child is using the prosthesis and is participating in the usual rough and tumble world of children.

The complications and problems of child amputees are also quite different from and vastly smaller in magnitude than those of adult amputees. The following categories of complications (Aitken and France 1953) are common to amputees of all ages: (1) scar formation, (2) spur formation, (3) neuromata, (4) short stumps, (5) bony overgrowth, (6) phantom limb, and (7) phantom pain.

Scar formation is not a problem, even in adults. In the last twenty years, giant steps have been taken in the area of prosthetic fittings, made possible primarily by the availability of new plastic materials that are more workable and less irritating to the stump. The classic amputation incisions and scars that were described after World War II have now been supplanted by prosthetic advancement. A good prosthetist can fit a socket regardless of scar placement. Spur formation is more a radiographic finding than a real problem. This usually — and frequently — occurs at the ends of bones. Again, advances in prosthetic materials and shapes have rendered this complication almost innocuous. Stump neuromata that were significant enough to necessitate further surgery occurred in 3.7 percent of children in a large series (Aitken and Frantz 1953).

Short stumps can be a problem in both children and adults. Despite prosthetic advancements, a stump that is too short to motorize the prosthesis is a problem. As mentioned earlier, an attempt should be made to salvage growth plates in children in order that the stump may continue to grow to an appropriate length. A stump that is too long can always be revised at maturity.

The bony overgrowth at the end of a stump is a little understood phenomenon that occurs in children but not in adults. Bony overgrowth occurs through a transected bone, not a disarticulation. The fibula and humerus are the bones most commonly affected. Surgical revision is necessary in approximately 6 percent of amputations.

Phantom limb is the perception that the limb is still present. This is best explained by the brain's continuing to perceive the limb as completely intact although it has been amputated. This is a condition that exists in most children up to about a year after amputation and then declines to a very small percentage. Again, the younger the child, the less time the brain has had to perceive the intact limb; therefore, the younger the child, the less the problem with a phantom limb. Phantom pain, on the other hand, is the phenomenon of pain in the amputated part. This is a serious problem in older amputees, but is practically never a problem in children.

PSYCHOSOCIAL ASPECTS

The vast majority of child amputees exhibit no anxiety or emotional dysfunction because of their amputation. Nevertheless, physicians and other health care workers should keep in mind that some children and their families do have problems, many of which are not easily voiced but may be brought out by counseling. In cases of traumatic amputation, both parents and child are overwhelmed by the suddenness and the extent of the loss. Their first response is "Why did this happen to us?" The treating physician has a key responsibility at this point. As well as managing the patient medically, the physician must also be attuned to these problems of psyche.

One of the most effective means of assisting parents and child are parent support groups or parent outreach groups (Chepolis and Thorp 1984; Clark, McCloskey, and Anderson 1977; Simons 1983; Sullivan and Celikyol 1976; Talbot and Solomon 1978). In questioning many parents, Suderman, Tervo, and Leszczynski (1982) found that most of them felt that the time they most needed emotional support was early on, when they felt the sense of loneliness the most severely. Parent support groups can supply both emotional stability and counseling in the early days after the child's injury. As in many pediatric conditions, parent and child are closely interwoven. If one does well, the other will probably do well. For this reason, it must be borne in mind that both must be treated.

Formal parent support groups are an integral part of any amputee clinic. Their purposes are manifold, but the foremost are to provide immediate support to the family and to provide a frame of reference for the future. For example, the parents of a normal six-year-old girl have a fairly good idea of what to expect when she reaches her sixteenth year. However, the parents of a six-year-old girl who has just lost her lower leg have no idea how this daughter will be as a sixteen-year-old. In these support groups, there are parents who have passed through this phase. They can be comforting and can provide a frame of reference for what to expect as the child grows older. The parent support networks are also beneficial for the dissemination of information regarding amputee programs such as skiing, camping, and so on. I emphasize that the leaders of the parent support groups should be lay parents, not physicians or even other health care workers. Naturally, medical personnel will be advisory to the group, but it is the parents' organization and they should determine the direction of the group's efforts.

While they are going through the difficult process of growing up, all children, normal or amputee, need love and acceptance by their parents, friends, and society; adventure and opportunities to explore the world; rebellion; privacy; achievement and a basis for self-esteem (Taylor 1970). The important point is that the child amputee has the same needs that normal children do. The way in which many of these needs are met will obviously be modified. Nevertheless, the same needs are present.

Parental love of the child and acceptance of the child's impairment are two very different things. For example, the parents may continue to love the child, but they may not be able to accept the limitations imposed on the child by the amputation. This can lead to parental discord that can also affect the child and the rest of the family. An example is the overly protective parent who feels that the child amputee has to be driven everywhere and prevented from participating in any physical activities. At the other extreme is the parent who feels that the child should be an "overachiever," and therefore encourages the child to participate in physical activity that is inappropriate, such as running five miles on an artificial limb. If both of these parent types are in the same family, there will be a problem. Again, parent support groups can often put a child's limitations in a proper perspective.

All of us who treat children must remember that they have a need for privacy, both personal and for their tangible possessions. Many amputee clinics tend to violate some of the principles of privacy by needlessly exposing children and their prostheses to other patients and parents in the clinic. They forget that there is a more important child attached to the amputated limb. Another point for medical personnel to remember is that self-esteem is very important to these children. Studies have shown that their confidence and self-esteem vary with their surroundings. For example, an amputee may feel quite comfortable sitting in school, where the major activity is verbal; however, the child is less confident in a marching band or on the playground. A study by Lyttle, Spencer, and Perry (1976) showed that patients were least confident when they were in a physician's office. Therefore, all of us should strive to emphasize how the whole patient is doing and not just "How is your leg?"

Children can often be helped by participating in patient support groups. These groups disseminate information, redirect goals for children, provide personal experience, serve as forums for the general exchange of ideas, and provide appropriate frames of reference for the future.

Overall, the incidence of depression and anxiety reactions is low in child amputees, but problems do occur among adolescent amputees (Schweitzer and Rosenbaum 1982). Many patients in this older group have had psychosocial difficulties in the past, such as family problems, school problems, including dropping out of school, loss of a job, or the like. Such patients do not have a strong support system. They are overly concerned about their future and exhibit more depression after the injury. A fair number of these patients may slip into substance abuse, which only accentuates their depression and anger.

Replantation in the lower extremity has had far different results than replantation in the upper extremity. According to Kleinert, Jablon, and Tsai (1980) the only indication for replantation in the lower extremity is a partial foot amputation in a child. However, upper extremity replantation, done on the basis of the appropriate indications, has had a success rate of approximately 90 percent. These data are based on the parameters of two-point discrimination, grip strength, range of motion, the absence of cold intolerance, and return to employment. The advent of external fixators such as the Hoffman Frame has also markedly advanced care of severely injured limbs with both bony and soft tissue damage. Undoubtedly, many injured lower extremities, particularly tibias, have been saved by the judicious use of these fixators.

SUMMARY

Following traumatic amputation, children do remarkably well with respect to both orthopedic function and psychosocial adjustment. As a general rule, younger children do better than older children. This rule that the younger the amputee, the better the result applies to patients in childhood through the third decade of life (the age of the largest war casualty group), through those in their early fifties (Parkes 1976) and into the elderly group (Caplan and Hackett 1963). Ninety percent of child amputees use their prosthesis. They seem to be more concerned with function than form, and are not overly concerned with their appearance or with exhibiting the prosthesis for others to see. Psychosocially, children and their families have needs during the period soon after the amputation when they face many questions concerning the future. This is often a time of depression and anger. Parent support groups and outreach groups are the best means of providing counseling and guidance. Medical workers such as psychologists and others are available for families who need more indepth help.

REFERENCES

Aitken, G. and C. Frantz. 1953. "The Juvenile Amputee." *Orthopedic Clinics of North America* 3:447.

Caplan, L. and T. Hackett. 1963. "Emotional Effects of Lower-Limb Amputation in the Aged." *New England Journal of Medicine* 269(22): 1166-1171.

Chepolis, L. and N. Thorp. 1984. "Networking Families in a Prosthetic Clinic for Children." *Inter-Clinic Information Bulletin* 19:80-82.

Clark, M., S. McCloskey, and L. Anderson. 1977. "Camp Workshop for Adolescent Amputees." *Inter-Clinic Information Bulletin* 16:(5-6):1-6.

Edelstein, J. 1985. "New Title, New Policy, New Outlook." *Journal of the Association of Children's Prosthetic-Orthotic Clinics* 20(3):33.

Kleinert, H., M. Jablon, and T. Tsai. 1980. "An Overview of Replantation and Results of 347 Replants in 245 Patients." *Journal of Trauma* 20:390-397.

Lyttle, D., D. Spencer, and R. Perry. 1976. "Satisfaction and Self-Esteem in Patients Attending a Juvenile Amputee Clinic." *Inter-Clinic Information Bulletin* 15(3-4):1-8.

Parkes, C. 1976. "The Psychological Reaction to Loss of a Limb: The First Year After Amputation." In J. G. Howell, ed. *Modern Perspectives in the Psychiatric Aspects of Surgery*. New York: Brunner/Mazel.

Schweitzer, I. and M. Rosenbaum. 1982. "Psychiatric Aspects of Replantation Surgery." *General Hospital Psychiatry* 4(4):271-279.

Simons, E. 1983. "An Evolutionary Perspective on the Development of a Parent Association: Child Amputee Support Society." *Inter-Clinic Information Bulletin* 18(3):13-16.

Suderman, V., R. Tervo, and J. Leszczynski. 1982. "Patient and Family Perspectives of a Juvenile Amputee Clinic." *Inter-Clinic Information Bulletin* 18(2):1-4.

Sullivan, R. and F. Celikyol. 1976. "An Ongoing Seminar for Parents of Amputee Children." *Inter-Clinic Information Bulletin* 15(5-6):9-14.

Talbot, D. and C. Solomon. 1978. "The Function of a Parent Group in the Adaptation to the Birth of a Limb-Deficient Child." *Inter-Clinic Information Bulletin* 17(1):9-10.

Taylor, I. W. 1970. "Psychological Needs of the Handicapped Child." *Inter-Clinic Information Bulletin* 9(8):9-17.

Tooms, R. 1980. "Amputations." In A. Edmonson and A. Crenshaw, eds. *Campbell's Operative Orthopaedics*, 6th ed. St. Louis: C. V. Mosby.

VanDerwerker, E. E., Jr. 1976. "A Brief Review of the History of Amputations and Prostheses." *Inter-Clinic Information Bulletin* 15(5-6):15-16.

Emotional Reactions
to the Loss of a Body Part

Rodman Gilder

Following amputation, a child often experiences anxiety, anger, shame, depressive affect, and even guilt. Although these emotions may be more or less repressed and otherwise defended against, the most fundamental and consistent is depressive affect, which is the natural reaction to a loss. This is true for any loss—loss of a loved one, loss of the expectation of life and growth, and loss of part of one's body.

Shame may be a prominent reaction to the loss of a body part. A visual change often seems to produce even more embarrassment than functional limitation. Shame is the emotional reaction to the realization that one is not living up to one's ego ideal. It has to do with a loss of self-esteem. Thus, along with the loss of a leg, for instance, the child is threatened with a painful loss of self-esteem and feelings of shame. Such feelings may be heavily defended against by denial and reaction formation—for example, the child may boast about the amputation and display the stump. In the short run, considering the severity of the loss, such behavior is not always maladaptive.

A child experiences the same dysphoric emotions in anticipation of the loss of a body part, but at this time the emphasis is on anxiety in anticipation of what is to come. This raises questions for staff and parents: When should the child be informed of the need for amputation, and how should the child be told? There are no pat answers, no assuredly helpful rules of thumb. Every case has to be considered individually. We have found, however, that it helps us gauge how

Rodman Gilder, MD, is Associate Clinical Professor in Psychiatry, College of Physicians and Surgeons, Columbia University, New York, NY.

© 1988 by The Haworth Press, Inc. All rights reserved.

to respond if we can find out just what the child is experiencing and what he or she anticipates, and if we then make clear to the child the reality that at least stands against any unwarranted fear.

Those who are close to the child, especially parents and hospital staff, may experience similar emotions and similar defenses. It seems that empathy is essential to understand what the child is experiencing and to help guide us in the care of the child. Yet the danger in overidentifying with the child and unconsciously taking on the child's emotions and defenses is that we can lose a certain detachment and objectivity. Ideally, we should be involved and objective at the same time — a tall order indeed.

An example of overidentification is the doctor who goes along with the child, pretends that everything is fine, denies his own depressive affect and feelings of shame, and desperately maintains a laughing front. The good side of this behavior is that it accentuates the positive, which, for a very brief time, can be helpful. The bad side is that the child's darker feelings of depression and anger are untouched and unexpressed, so that the child feels left alone and isolated.

One way to find out a child's feelings after an amputation has been done is to ask about the phantom limb. Almost all patients seem to feel a phantom — only 2 percent of amputees claim no phantom at all. Perception of the phantom limb may last for months and then tends to disappear gradually. It is often worth establishing with the child the presence of the phantom limb and to help the child through the shame barrier — that is, that it is not crazy and that it is all right to have a phantom of the amputated limb. Patient's emotional states can affect the size, shape, position, and painfulness of the phantom. Caregivers can learn something about the patient by eliciting a running account of the phantom.

This can be illustrated by the case of an eighteen-year-old boy who barely survived an automobile accident. Both of his legs were crushed and his left leg had to be amputated below the knee. The boy had been a boxer and a runner. At school he was known as a fighter who fought to win. After the amputation, he first suffered severe phantom pain. He said that it felt as if the phantom foot were held curled in a vise, the leg straight out and immovable. The phantom expressed how he felt: frustrated, enraged, and unable to change his situation. During psychoanalytically oriented psychotherapy, the patient was able to work with his feelings, thoughts, fantasies, and dreams. He was able to work through to a gradual and partial acceptance of his amputation. Along with this, his phantom changed — the pain disappeared and the phantom became shorter, more relaxed, and more movable.

Psychiatric evaluation and treatment are indicated when a patient's emotions interfere with the smooth process of recovery and rehabilitation. This is obvious, for example, when a child is angry, oppositional, in much more pain than is warranted. A more hidden situation, which the staff is more likely to miss, occurs when the child is quiet and cooperative, but manifests depression by not eating well, not sleeping well, or by withdrawal. In this instance, dialogue may follow a pattern something like the following: "How are you doing today, Johnny?" "Fine." "You look great." Silence or, again, "Fine." Such children can use help with some of their not-so-fine feelings. Mothers and nurses are apt to be more aware of children's depressive affect than doctors, who do not spend as much time with the children.

It can be extremely useful for families to have contact with other families whose children have undergone amputations, which can occur, for example, in parent support groups. Parents and their families are impressed and reassured by other children who have successfully negotiated their rehabilitation with an effective prosthesis.

In conclusion, improvements in surgical techniques and rehabilitation, including advances in prosthetic devices and early ambulation, have gone a long way to compensate not only for the loss of a limb, but for the idea of the loss, and to mitigate the disturbing emotional reactions. However, children who have had a limb amputated know that the loss has, in fact, occurred. Although they may hide their feelings, those feelings can be strong enough to interfere with recovery, and therefore should be dealt with. The goal is to help patients work through the mourning for what they have lost so that they can free themselves to proceed with rehabilitation and with life.

Reaction of Children and Adolescents to Amputation

Joan Kaiser

The amputation of a limb, at any age and for any reason, is a difficult experience, but it is especially devastating for an older child or adolescent. In some instances, the options are amputation or limb salvage surgery, and if limb salvage has been expected but is not technically possible, the amputation is that much more traumatic.

Adolescents are in a period of transition in which they experience intense physical, emotional, and social changes and face the developmental challenges that are part of their passage to adulthood. Even for healthy children, adolescence can be a difficult period, but once the issue arises of the necessity to amputate an extremity, the developmental issues can become overwhelming.

The developmental tasks of adolescence have two major aspects. First, youths emerge from adolescence with a sense of themselves as unique, sexual individuals; second, they use that identity to become independent persons. The sense of self needs to be derived from within and independently of the family unit. Teenagers automatically begin to address developmental issues as they experience physical growth and change, intellectual development, and psychosocial maturation. Hormonal changes trigger the adolescent growth spurt and the development of secondary sexual characteristics. These changes become important for shaping the body image of adolescents.

As mental maturation occurs, adolescents, by age thirteen or so, have acquired the mental operations for adult thinking. In contrast

---

Joan Kaiser, RN, MA, Staff Development, Good Samaritan Hospital, Suffern, NY.

© 1988 by The Haworth Press, Inc. All rights reserved.   *15* to younger children, they are able to reason about things beyond their actual experience or knowledge and to consider things that are believed to be contrary to fact. Their emerging capacity for introspection is also important. Successful maturation leaves the adolescent with a sold sense of self-esteem. Psychosocial development parallels the development of self-esteem and body image.

Successful formation of a sense of identity, then, includes acceptance of body changes, separation from parents, establishment of close peer relationships, formation of a comfortable sexual identity, and selection of career goals. After examining the developmental issues of adolescence, the devastating impact of illness and amputation becomes clear. The adolescent's reaction to radical surgery is commonly manifested by the fear of pain, mutilation, abandonment, and death. In this context, there may be an actual feeling of relief after the surgery.

In terms of developmental tasks, at a time when physical attractiveness and function are essential to the development of a healthy self-concept, illness and mutilating surgery can halt developmental progress. *All* developmental tasks are affected, not just the acceptance of the physical body and the changes it normally undergoes.

The issue of independence from parents is delayed, since any severely ill person must at times rely on family for care, including support and companionship while in the hospital and assistance with necessities like transportation to and from the hospital or physician's office for treatment or follow-up care. Emancipated teenagers may need to move back home if they become too ill to manage alone. Absence from school, another area of concern, decreases cognitive stimulation and growth and entails a loss of opportunity for socialization with peers.

Hospitalization and treatments further separate these adolescents from their friends, interfering with peer relationships. This can be mitigated by the use of flexible visiting hours to accommodate school and work schedules. However, some teenagers and children voluntarily withdraw from their friends, anticipating rejection because of the way surgery or chemotherapy, if it has been necessary to treat cancer, has altered their appearance.

One method of increasing socialization and providing patients with a peer support structure is by the formation of a sharing or support group within the hospital. Participation in such groups helps the patients realize they are not alone, that others are coping with similar problems of amputation, radical surgery, and cancer. This is especially useful for out-of-town patients who have been referred to a big-city hospital for treatment and thus are distant from their normal support systems.

Another factor to consider among the effects of amputation is, of course, the compromise of the teenager's functional status. This can necessitate changes in present life-style, as well as the need to reconsider and, perhaps, to alter vocational and life goals.

The adolescent's adaptation to amputation is influenced by many interrelated factors, including the individual's background, ability to cope, interests, and available outside support. Walters (1981) has described a four-phase process in the adjustment of an adolescent or older child to amputation of an extremity. These phases are impact, retreat, acknowledgment, and reconstruction.

IMPACT

This phase is initiated when an adolescent learns that the treatment plan includes amputation. Adolescents who are under the age of consent must be included in the treatment plan, actual treatment decisions, and follow-up. At some institutions, adolescents are required to co-sign consent forms as evidence of their active involvement in their treatment; this is known as assent. Although adolescents' signatures are not legally binding, this practice allows the patients some control and reinforces awareness among the health care team of the adolescent's "vested interest" in the treatment.

Amputation may be the only treatment available, as in cases of severe trauma or nonresectable tumors. Amputation may also be offered if other procedures have failed—for example, if infection has set in after a limb salvage procedure or if it is revealed that a tumor has not been completely resected.

Although adolescents can understand that amputation is necessary in order for them to survive, their intense sense of physical appearance is felt more strongly. Despair, discouragement, passive acceptance, or angry denial may result. Although denial may be seen as a pathological defense in the resolution of conflict, it is a normal defense that is temporarily and appropriately used at the time of diagnosis. Most patients will vacillate between denial and acceptance throughout the course of their illness. Amputees, however, are less likely to deny their illness for an extended time. One study of children's adjustment to limb amputation showed that their primary response is depression, followed by expressions of rejection of the amputation and fear.

During the impact phase, patients require support and education. Teenagers are risk-takers, but they must be helped to understand that if they accept no treatment, their lives are at risk. Once they understand the risks of treatment versus those of no treatment, they are more likely to cooperate and accept the necessary decision. In addition to reinforcement of the physician's explanation of the need for amputation, preoperative teaching should focus on exactly what will happen during surgery and what it will feel like after surgery.

Preoperative teaching for the younger child should include play therapy, in which the child has the opportunity to see a doll with the same limb amputated at the same level that theirs will be, and to touch the stump. Preoperative physical therapy can be used to provide information on the rehabilitation program that will be followed and to begin crutch training, preliminary instruction on stump care, and to teach conditioning exercises. All of this, of course, must be tailored to the needs of each patient and how much information he or she is ready to hear. A preoperative visit with another patient who has undergone amputation is extremely helpful, although many patients prefer to have the visit once the amputation is over.

Preoperative evaluation for both patient and family by the medical social worker is important. Social work intervention includes support, exploration of feelings about diagnosis and treatment, and help in dealing with the hospital system. Members of the family may understand the implications of the disease more fully than the patient does, and will therefore be more responsive to help from the social worker.

Because a common reaction of family members is to attempt to protect one another from painful feelings, it is important to leave open the lines of communication within the family system. If the patient expresses sadness, anger, or depression, the family should be encouraged to allow him or her to do so fully and to understand that this is healthy and normal. Silence and denial on the family's part will feed into the denial, isolation, and displacement of feelings in both the patient and the family.

RETREAT

As the reality of amputation becomes apparent, the patient enters the second phase of adjustment, retreat. During this phase, the patient mourns for the loss of a limb, experiencing the acute grief of all people dealing with loss. The young person's grieving is for the lost limb and also for the loss of anticipation of the self as a complete adult. This phase is characterized by somatic and emotional reactions and by changes in behavior, including anxiety, tension, depression, fear, guilt, anger, lethargy, dependency, and regressive behavior, as well as anorexia and weight loss. The patient may refuse to look at or touch the stump.

The body image changes resulting from amputation are obvious and must be discussed with the child or adolescent. The patient will never be the same as before. Many adolescents have stated that the experience of being diagnosed and treated for cancer has caused them to feel different from their peers, not only because of the body changes but also because of feelings of accelerated maturity. Verbalization plays a part in successful grieving, which results in acceptance of the loss and relinquishment of the hope of retrieving the lost object.

After the amputation, the patient may be angry and may direct this anger at the health care team. The staff should not react with defensiveness or hostility. Adolescents need to be informed that the health care team understands how angry and upset they must be and that the staff is willing to listen to them talk about their anger.

Adolescents may also feel guilty—"bad things happen to bad people." If, for example, the amputation is necessary because of cancer, patients may believe that if they had not ignored early symptoms the tumor might have been caught sooner and amputation would not have been necessary. Patients may also dwell on the pain and problems they have brought to their families.

Health care team objectives focus on reinforcing amputees' strengths and encouraging them to do as much for themselves as they can. It is important for amputees to perceive themselves realistically, and the staff should foster hope for the patient and family by reinforcing the fact that after the physical therapy program, the patient will function independently and well—how well, of course is based on the level of the amputation.

ACKNOWLEDGMENT

In this, the third phase of adjustment, patients are incorporating their changed physical appearance into their body image. Signs that a teenager has accepted the amputation include referring to the amputated extremity as a stump and expressing willingness to participate in the care and exercise program.

RECONSTRUCTION

During this phase of adjustment, rehabilitation is in full swing, prosthesis training has begun, patients' activities of daily living are worked out, their career goals are evaluated, and developmental tasks are addressed anew. At this point, the adolescent can think of how to deal with the reactions of others to the surgery.

This phase may be prolonged because many amputees must complete several months of postoperative chemotherapy before receiving a permanent prosthesis. This is because stump size will fluctuate during chemotherapy.

Reconstruction can be facilitated if the health care team encourages self-care and management, provides honest and accurate information, arranges treatments so that the patient can attend school as often as possible, and supports the patient's reengagement with peers.

For the younger child, reengagement may in some ways be more difficult than for the adolescent. After amputation, the young child reenters the community, which includes family, peer groups, and school, with many misgivings and feeling different from his or her friends. For a child, alopecia, weight loss, and amputation are frightening changes in body image. Amputation requires a particularly difficult and strenuous rehabilitation period, during which the child must make emotional and physical adjustments. Without help in these areas, a child risks becoming withdrawn and isolated from the peer group and may regress to dependent, infantile behavior within the family. Children must be allowed to express fears about going home to friends and, in relation to their own and their friends' anxiety, may need help in handling first encounters with them.

In conclusion, children and adolescents who have undergone amputation are at risk for developmental delay. Thus, it is essential that those who provide care for these patients have an understanding of developmental issues and how they affect the grieving and adaptational processes. This can help diminish some of the conflicts that inevitably arise.

REFERENCE

Walters, J. 1981. "Coping with a Leg Amputation." American Journal of Nursing 81:1349-1352.

Amputation and the Reconstruction of Congenital Lesions

David Price Roye, Jr.

Several severe congenital deficiencies of the lower extremities can sometimes be best reconstructed by amputation and prosthetic rehabilitation. The diagnostic categories that are primarily involved are (1) proximal femoral focal deficiency, (2) absence of the tibia, (3) absence of the fibula, and (4) severe shortening. Elective amputation may be recommended in other circumstances, but it is this group of lesions that most frequently gives rise to the situation in which parents must be advised that surgical ablation of part of the limb is necessary.

A proximal femoral focal deficiency is a hypoplasia of the proximal femur that encompasses a spectrum from a short femur with a stable hip articulation to an extremely short femur with no development of the hip joint at all. Aitken (1969) has categorized them into types A, B, C, and D. A is the simple shortening type and D is the most severe type, without hip joint. In the most severe forms, lengthening will not be possible because there is severe hypoplasia of tissues in the thigh, including the neurovascular bundles. The attempt to stretch these structures leads to pain or vascular compromise, which is not acceptable. The unstable hip articulation also contraindicates lengthening. All of this means that if the limb is left alone, the foot will ultimately be at a level close to the knee of the opposite normal limb. A large, heavy lift or a rather complicated prosthesis could be used, but the cosmetic and functional results are not good. A below-knee type of prosthesis with the foot in equinus can be used, but in this technique, the "knees" are at very different

David Price Roye, Jr., MD, is Assistant Professor of Orthopedic Surgery, College of Physicians and Surgeons, Columbia University, New York, NY.

© 1988 by The Haworth Press, Inc. All rights reserved.

23

levels. Once these problems are understood, the solution of amputation does not seem as radical.

The hip is stabilized surgically if possible. The foot is amputated
through its midportion, leaving the calcaneus and heel pad if possible, or at least the heel pad. If the entire hind foot cannot be sal-
vaged because of deformity, some modification of the Symes amputation can usually be performed. Eventually the knee is fused,
thus allowing the use of a relatively normal above-knee prosthesis,
which will give a good appearance and will place the knee articulation on the affected side at the same level as the contralateral normal
knee.

When the problem is an absent fibula or tibia, there is a deformed
foot with an unstable ankle that frequently defies reconstruction.
When a stable foot cannot be obtained, amputation is again recommended. The patient can then be fitted with a below-knee prosthesis
that has an excellent cosmetic appearance. If the deformed foot is
maintained, prosthetic fitting is complicated. The resulting prosthesis is likely to be bulky and not be nearly so cosmetic.

Parents whose infant is facing elective amputation for reconstruction of a congenital lesion have a different sort of decision to make
than the parents of children who have a malignancy or other life-
threatening illness. If the child has a sarcoma that cannot be reconstructed or has a terrible infection and amputation is recommended,
the decision does not involve a great deal of difficulty. However,
when the foot for which the surgeon is recommending amputation
looks normal, the decision is very difficult. The major issues here
are not really the technical aspects of patient management. The
problem is presenting the information and alternatives to parents in
a way that allows them to make an informed decision. The difficulties are several:

1. The parents are already facing the fact that their infant is not
   perfect and has a major congenital deformity. As they mourn
   the loss of that perfection, they must face the necessity of
   making other decisions involving loss, such as amputation of a
   limb. Even though it may be "only a foot" that will be ab-
   lated, this is an extremely difficult decision for parents to face.
2. Parents are distraught about their new baby's deformity. They

may feel that they created the deformity and are contributing to the child's trouble by requesting or allowing amputation.

3. The affected foot often looks quite normal. Thus, parents are understandably reluctant to allow its removal. It is not uncommon for them to have an unrealistic expectation that something miraculous may occur to allow limb salvage, and this adds to their reluctance to allow amputation.

The solutions are not always straightforward, but in general we start by carefully outlining all of the management plans and the reasons behind them. Often this information must be repeated several times before all of it is absorbed. We recommend genetic counseling to round out parents' understanding and to allay their feelings of guilt. We recommend family counseling to allow them to deal with their feelings about the deformity and the recommended treatment. We also ask parents to talk to other parents who have gone through the same dilemma, having found that this is reassuring to the parents. Finally, we ask them to see a young amputee. This last step, I believe, is one of the most helpful. Seeing a young, vigorous child successfully using a prosthesis can be quite convincing.

All of this should be accomplished during the first year of the child's life. Most pediatric orthopedists feel that these amputations are most safely performed when the child is about twelve months of age: structures are larger and the child's developmental status is clearer than at earlier ages. In addition, prosthetic rehabilitation can begin close to the normal age for walking, at twelve to twenty-four months. We also believe that children do not have a sense of loss from the amputation when it is performed at this early age.

REFERENCE

Aitken, G. T. 1969. "Proximal Femoral Focal Deficiency." In C. A. Swinyard, ed. *Limb Development and Deformities: Problems of Evaluation and Rehabilitation*. Springfield, IL: Charles C Thomas.

II. LOSS OF A PERFECT CHILD

Loss of the "Perfect" Child and Ethical Decision Making: Miguel's Story

Zola D. Golub

An infant boy is delivered normally at term, but he is abnormal. His head is of normal size, but he has a broad forehead, wide-set eyes, and a small jaw. He has multiple clefts in his tongue and a cleft soft palate. All of his extremities are significantly foreshortened; the joints look abnormal. He has seven fingers on one hand, six on the other, and seven toes on each foot. He has bilateral club feet and his hips are dislocated.

The infant's mother, a woman in her late thirties, is separated from the infant's father, who lives in another country; their three other children live with her. She lives with her sister's family—there are fifteen in all—in a four-room apartment. Her income consists of welfare payments. When the mother sees the newborn, she immediately recognizes his physical appearance as being "just like" that of her daughter, born three years earlier, who had lived at home until her death.

Zola D. Golub, MEd, RN, is Instructor, Neonatal Intensive Care Unit, Columbia-Presbyterian Medical Center, New York, NY.

© 1988 by The Haworth Press, Inc. All rights reserved.

27

This infant, Miguel, is admitted to our neonatal intensive care unit for further evaluation of his abnormalities. The orthopedist believes that with multiple surgical procedures and long-term rehabilitation, Miguel's limb abnormalities can be ameliorated. The geneticist establishes that Miguel has normal chromosomes and finds the physical defects to be consistent with a particular congenital syndrome. The prognosis for infants with this syndrome is variable and difficult to predict, but the geneticist explains that it is correlated with the extent of the neurological damage that also is generally associated with this syndrome. A CT scan reveals various midline brain abnormalities, including a large posterior cyst communicating with the fourth ventricle of the brain. Miguel's electroencephalogram is grossly abnormal.

Consistent with the severity of Miguel's congenital brain defects, on about his second or third day of life he begins to experience six to eight episodes a day in which he stops breathing, turns blue, and requires significant resuscitative efforts to revive him. The neurologist believes that these episodes are manifestations of seizure activity and suggests anticonvulsant medication. With the medication, Miguel has significantly fewer episodes—one or two every couple of days.

Miguel requires oxygen administered via a headbox to maintain adequate oxygenation of his tissues. As a consequence of his brain abnormalities, he is unable to suck or swallow; therefore, he requires frequent suctioning to remove secretions from his mouth and throat. A nasogastric feeding tube is passed through Miguel's mouth and into his stomach to allow him to receive formula slowly and continuously. Miguel's mother comes to visit him frequently. The physicians fully explain Miguel's condition to her. She tells the physicians and nurses that she wants her son to live and that she wants everything possible done to help him to do so.

To those who care for him, Miguel is not a beautiful or appealing child. Apart from his physical deformities, he is irritable, often making facial grimaces and crying a great deal. At other times he sleeps. He does not display any periods of quiet wakefulness or observation of his environment. He does not interact with those who are caring for him. The nurses and physicians on our neonatal unit express the expected continuum of emotion and opinion about

Miguel: disgust, pity, avoidance, active resentment, and caring compassion. Some believe that his mother wants the infant to be treated vigorously because she either does not comprehend or is denying the severity of his physical and mental abnormalities and the burdens that caring for him will entail. Some are deeply saddened and disturbed by the situation.

By the time her son is one week old, Miguel's mother displays symptoms of significant depression. She is unable to sleep or eat well; she reports recurrent memories of the death of Miguel's sister, "who was so like him." She also expresses severe guilt feelings related to her fear of being asked for "permission" to let the baby die. She believes that the physicians do not understand her desire to have everything possible done for her son or her wish to learn whatever is necessary to care for him appropriately at home, even for just a few months.

The processes and principles of ethical decision making involve issues that are complex and profound. How should we proceed to decide about Miguel's care? Physicians, nurses, and others who are caring for Miguel are keenly aware that we are dealing with emotionally charged questions with high stakes: the life or death of an infant. Miguel's mother is deeply troubled; she has already experienced the tragic loss of her infant daughter. All of us are stressed by the fact that Miguel confronts us with these decisions. What would Miguel choose for himself, we wonder. We are forced to render a decision by proxy for someone who is incompetent and has never been competent. We realize the potential for significant disagreement and conflict of interest.

What sorts of treatment ought to be offered to this child? Our sense of justice demands that the decisions regarding Miguel's care not depend on which particular physicians and nurses happen, by chance, to be charged with this care. What principles should guide this decision? What process ought to be set in motion when an infant like Miguel is admitted to a neonatal intensive care unit?

A close examination of these questions reveals that two different kinds of issues are confronting us. The first issues are substantive. What is the right thing to do in this case? Should Miguel receive every treatment modality that is available? Should he undergo neurosurgery? Orthopedic surgery? Or would we be inflicting needless pain and suffering on an infant who will never be able to understand or appreciate our efforts? What about the expense? Should Miguel's mother be taught to care for him at home? Should she be taught how to do suctioning? CPR? How to operate a cardiac monitor? Should Miguel be placed in an institution? Are we underestimating Miguel's potential? Can we anticipate or predict the powerful effects of his mother's love and determination on her son? The second set of issues is procedural. Who should make the decisions, and by what process? Does Miguel's mother alone have the right to decide? Should Miguel's father be consulted? Do the health care professionals have any say?

Having separated these two types of issues in an effort to clarify the outstanding decisions, it is important to emphasize that within the realm of ethical decision making, the "what" and "how" are intimately linked. Decisions about either affect both.

In an ideal world, decision makers would be wise and astute. They would possess expertise about all of the medical facts of the case, and the implications of these facts for diagnosis and prognosis would then be unmistakable. Decision makers would be fully enlightened and compassionate about the personal aspects of the case — the family situation and the cultural connotations. They would be learned and erudite about the principles and processes that lead to consistent and just decisions. These decision makers would be emotionally mature and rock stable, and would have all the time they needed to consider the myriad of complex data involved in any case.

In reality, perhaps the best that can be done is for the physicians and other health team members who are caring for Miguel communicate with and listen to Miguel's mother with sympathy and sensitivity. We may encourage her to seek the advice of people who are significant to her — perhaps a member of the clergy or a family member. We who are caring for Miguel may seek the advice of our ethics committee. Recalling the multifaceted dimensions of the issues here, it is clear that no one person should be asked to bear the full weight of the decisions and their consequences.

Parents are the primary decision makers for their children. This right is an extension of the discretionary decision-making power and authority that is granted to parents by our society. One can assume that the parents will make a decision that is in the child's best interest. (The fact that a few parents will make a decision that is clearly not in a child's best interest must not compel us to deny the decision-making right to the majority of parents, who are genuinely concerned with their children's well-being. To do so would be analogous to eliminating the jury system because a jury occasionally convicts an innocent person.) It is parents who have the most to gain as well as the most to lose as a consequence of any decision regarding the medical treatment of their child.

Physicians and other health care professionals who are caring for the child must also be included in the process. They are, after all, the most expert in the medical realm and the most experienced concerning diagnosis, prognosis, and possible treatment. Moreover, an ethics committee, consisting of a multidisciplinary team educated in the rigorous thinking processes involved in ethical decision making, can be valuable as a resource to both parents and caregivers. The ethics committee may suggest alternative solutions or new ideas to consider. In addition, the committee may act as a safeguard in the rare instance that primary decision makers arrive at a decision that is clearly not in the child's best interest.

In our experience, knowledge of the existence of an ethics committee gives attending physicians, residents, and nurses "permission" to raise, examine, and discuss the potential ethical issues involved in an infant's care. This creates an atmosphere that is conducive to the decision-making process. As more ethical issues, principles, and concepts are discussed on a unit, the health care team becomes more knowledgeable about ethics and more comfortable with the decision-making process. The existence of an ethics committee has had a significant impact on the frequency and the quality of the discussions that nurses, physicians, and others on our unit have with parents. Increasingly effective communication and decision making concerning these hard choices is taking place.

We must remember that even given the best of circumstances — intelligent, knowledgeable, emotionally stable parents and health care providers who communicate with one another effectively and sensitively — even in these circumstances, the hard cases involving infants like Miguel, whose prognosis is unknown and whose best interest is difficult to discern, will leave us feeling, in part, confused, hurt, frustrated, dissatisfied, and anguished even after we have come to a resolution. Normally we try to avoid the situations that even at best leave us feeling uncomfortable. But as responsible caregivers we must not avoid these decisions because to do so forces a decision by default or by chance. Clearly, such a decision is unacceptable. Therefore, we need to continue to discuss these difficult questions. In so doing, we support and nurture each other as we strive to learn the processes and the principles that will lead us to just, ethical decision making with our patients and their families.

III. CHRONIC LOSS AND DISABILITY

Seeking Significance

Kenneth J. Doka

It has long been recognized that those facing personal finitude often search for meaning and significance in their lives. In the face of death, we seek affirmation that our lives have had purpose. For example, Erikson (1950) characterized the last developmental stage as "ego integrity versus despair." Erikson's central concept is that as elderly people recognize that they are near the end of life, they begin a process of life review. To Erikson, that review concludes successfully if the individual can affirm that his or her life has been worthwhile. The underlying assumption is that in this search for significance, individuals seek to integrate their life's goals, values, and experiences so that they can assert that their life has made sense and that they have left a legacy, however small.

This theme is reflected in a number of other concepts, including Butler's (1963) "life review," Marshall's (1980) "awareness of finitude," and Lifton and Olson's (1974) "symbolic immortality," which includes the notion that this quest for meaning also entails a

Kenneth J. Doka, PhD, is Professor of Gerontology, Graduate School, College of New Rochelle, New Rochelle, NY.

© 1988 by The Haworth Press, Inc. All rights reserved.

33

desire to live on in one's creations and descendants as well as in a transcendental manner.

Studies of elderly populations indicate that members of this group do, in fact, review their lives to find significance (Riley 1968). Evidence of this same life review process has been found in younger dying populations (Noyes and Klett 1977), suggesting that the process is related to the awareness of finitude rather than age per se.

A parallel process has also been observed in the bereaved. The resolution of grief is often facilitated when the bereaved can affirm that the deceased's life had meaning and purpose. With an adult, this is usually not difficult. In developing that sense of significance, one can assess the person's achievements, offspring, personal triumphs, participation in great historical events, legacies, and impact on others. When a child dies, the situation is often more problem-filled. The child's potential may seem unfulfilled and wasted. It may be difficult to find affirmation of significance in a child's accomplishments, and harder still in an infant's. A child's achievements within a limited life span may simply highlight the tragedy and loss of death.

This failure to find significance may complicate the resolution of grief, intensifying feelings of anger, guilt, and resentment. The bereaved's inability to affirm a realistic sense of significance can lead to idealization of the dead child that complicates relationships with spouse, surviving children, and friends. It is essential, then, that grief counselors, clergy, and medical caregivers be sensitive to parents' need to find significance in the life of their deceased child and in their relationship with that child.

This article explores some of the ways in which that search can be accomplished. Although much of the information may be relevant to situations of sudden death, the focus is on the chronically ill child. I will not directly address the issues raised by perinatal deaths or particular circumstances such as child or adolescent suicide. Again, many of the same concerns would apply, but the special nature of such deaths merits separate discussion. Finally, I will not focus on the ways in which children themselves may search for that significance as they undergo their life review.

FINDING SIGNIFICANCE

Parents search for significance in their child's life in many ways. They will wish to talk about and review the child's life. The resolution of grief will be facilitated if they assert that the child's life, however short, had meaning. This resolution is often complicated by the conspiracy of silence that surrounds the child's memory. Significant others, seeing the parents' pain, feeling inadequate to discuss it, or feeling threatened by the death, may avoid discussion of the deceased child.

It is important for the parents to have opportunities to remember and to explore the meaning of the child's life. This can be facilitated in various ways. Those who were involved in some way with the deceased child may wish to share with the parents the ways in which the child's life or manner of death influenced them. One mother of a seven-year-old leukemia victim remembered how touched she was when a chaplain indicated the many ways in which her son had changed his ministry. Incidents or events that occurred during the child's hospitalization and that reflected the child's nature can often be of great value to the parents. One mother I know still treasures a letter from a hospice nurse that graphically describes the concern that her dying daughter had, even in the last days of her life, for other families and patients.

Medical staff can greatly facilitate the quest for significance. Through sensitivity to the underlying dynamics of this search for meaning, as well as the other dynamics of the family's values and system, and through their interaction with the hospital, medical staff can share with parents their own stories of the child's struggle, the child's impact on themselves and others, and the family's experiences. Medical staff may also wish to share what they have learned through the course of treating the child's illness that might assist other patients suffering from the same disease. This has to be done carefully, personally, and with warmth. An overly clinical, hurried, or objective discussion may suggest that the child was simply an experiment and that the value of the child's life lay only in his or her death. If the child had a long illness and hospitalization, I strongly suggest that at least one member of the staff attend the funeral. This, too, affirms the child's special significance.

Autopsies and organ donations can also help. One can extend Lifton and Olson's (1974) consideration of the modes of symbolic immortality—the ways in which a person lives on—to include a medical mode in which a person lives on in the enhanced or saved life of others. Sensitivity must be shown in the timing, selection of the person to make the request, and the phrasing of the request itself. And staff should quickly respect the parents' right of refusal. Although parents may appreciate the opportunity to find a sense of significance in organ donation or autopsy, it may also be seen as just one last assault on their child. A few meaningful gestures can enhance the therapeutic value of such actions. Nagy (1985) has described a program in one hospital in which there is a memorial service for all those who have donated bodies in the past six months. At that hospital, the medical library also has a special volume, exquisitely crafted and prominently displayed, that lists the names of donors.

Funeral directors can play an important role, since funeral rituals can have significant value. Although it is not the purpose of this article to review the role of the funeral in the resolution of grief, a few points seem especially relevant to this discussion. The funeral can provide opportunities for kin and friends to support the family by demonstrating and sharing the ways in which the child affected their lives. Often the very presence of these people—especially the child's peers, teachers, and other significant persons in the child's life—bears witness to the importance and value of the child's life. Teachers can encourage the attendance of staff and students and can help to prepare students and their families for the event.

The funeral can also provide a focal point for other acts that may affirm that meaning. It may be helpful for the parents to consider special scholarship funds or contributions that might perpetuate the child's memory. For example, one school used contributions in memory of a thirteen-year-old girl for a trophy case that would house all trophies for women's sports. Contributions should focus on things that are relevant, tangible, attractive, and that can be recognized by some sort of plaque or similar remembrance. (In one case, a parent of modest means was outraged when a priest, trying to be sensitive to her financial distress, suggested that her proffered contribution be used for some badly needed doormats.)

Following the funeral, parents will still need to discuss the impact of the child's life. Opportunities to consider that impact on family or community will facilitate grief resolution. Often, parental activities and personal growth will contribute to that sense of significance. Organizations such as Compassionate Friends or Mothers Against Drunk Driving (MADD) allow parents to reach out to others or to help pass socially beneficial legislation that will posthumously perpetuate the child's contribution and memory.

Private quests may also be of value. For example, the mother of one fourteen-year-old who committed suicide now frequently lectures to teachers' groups, PTAs, and school assemblies. Other parents have independently lobbied for the passage of new laws, worked toward the enactment of new safety regulations, or done research on important issues that relate in some way to their child's life or death. These quests should be discouraged only when they are clearly misguided, inappropriately focused, become personal vendettas, or have other deleterious effects.

Other activities such as compiling albums, writing journals or remembrances, or editing a film or cassette of the child's life can also assist parents in the search for significance. Some such works may even become substantial legacies. Long after their lives ended, John Guenther, Jr. and Eric Lund are still remembered through books written by their parents (Guenther 1953; Lund 1974).

The second goal of a life review process is to assist parents to perceive and affirm that the quality of their child's life, however short and constrained, was as high as possible. This is an affirmation of the parents' roles and relationship. The activities they enjoyed, the time they spent, the kindness and gifts they experienced, the struggle they shared, can be reviewed to facilitate that affirmation. Although reassurances by others, particularly medical staff, may alleviate guilt, parents need opportunities to express that guilt as well, as the range of emotions and actions that they experience. Activities such as participation in the care of the child (Hamovitch 1964) or in planning meaningful personalized rituals (Doka 1984) can enhance that role. Autopsies, too, may resolve lingering questions and help resolve guilt.

In the final analysis, the death of a child affronts our sense of order and justice. The death of a child conveys a sense of unfulfilled promise. But a human being has lived — for an hour, for a day, for ten years, and that life affords an opportunity to develop a realistic sense of the child's significance that will facilitate the resolution of grief.

REFERENCES

Butler, R. 1963. "The Life Review: An Interpretation of Reminiscence in the Aged." *Psychiatry* 26(1):65-76.

Doka, K. J. 1984. "Expectations of Death, Participation in Funeral Rituals, and Grief Adjustment." *Omega* 15:119-129.

Erikson, E. 1950. *Childhood and Society.* New York: W. W. Norton.

Guenther, J. 1953. *Death Be Not Proud.* New York: Random House.

Hamovitch, M. 1964. *The Parent and the Fatally Ill Child.* Duarte, CA: City of Hope Medical Center.

Lifton, R. J. and G. Olson. 1974. *Living and Dying.* New York: Bantam Books.

Lund, D. 1974. *Eric.* New York: Harper and Row.

Marshall, V. 1980. *Last Chapters: A Sociology of Aging and Dying.* Monterey, CA: Brooks/Cole.

Nagy, F. 1985. "A Model for a Donated Body Program in a School of Medicine." *Death Studies* 9:245-251.

Noyes, R. and R. Klett. 1977. "Panoramic Memory: A Response to the Threat of Death." *Omega* 8:181-194.

Riley, M. W. 1968. *Aging and Society.* New York: Russell Sage.

Pediatric Orthopedics:
Dealing with Loss
and Chronic Sorrow

Penelope R. Buschman

Over the years, as I have worked with chronically ill and disabled children and their families, I have become aware of these families' need to confront and deal with the feelings of loss and sadness that periodically come to the surface. Families do this at various times and in different ways as their children grow. Two vignettes from my clinical practice illustrate this phenomenon.

JERRY

Twelve-year-old Jerry is a developmentally delayed child with neurofibromatosis, which was diagnosed when he was two years old, and congenital scoliosis. His family includes his mother and father, both in their late thirties, a sixteen-year-old sister, his paternal grandparents, and an aunt. The sister, Dorothy, is treated for rheumatoid arthritis, which was diagnosed when she was three years old. Jerry was referred to me four years ago because of his depression and chronic anorexia. At that time, his family was both fatigued and discouraged. Since then, he and his family have been seen in treatment and for consultation.

In May 1984, as Jerry's scoliosis was growing worse and his day-to-day functioning was diminishing, his family decided to have the scoliosis corrected surgically, believing that such intervention

Penelope R. Buschman, RN, MS, is Assistant Professor of Clinical Nursing, School of Nursing, Columbia University, New York, NY. She is also Administrative Nurse Clinician, The Presbyterian Hospital in New York.

© 1988 by The Haworth Press, Inc. All rights reserved.

would improve Jerry's lung capacity and long-term outlook. This decision was contrary to the advice of the child's pediatrician, who recommended that no surgery be attempted.

While the parents gathered data about the surgery, its great risks, and the subsequent care Jerry would need, they (especially the mother) began to deal with the possibility of losing their child. At this time, they began to talk about their disappointment in Jerry's developmental achievements and his inability to contribute to the family in an age-appropriate manner. Recognizing the risks and the possibility of losing Jerry reactivated old feelings of loss and hurt that had been deeply buried.

Jerry survived the enormously complex two-stage surgery and is again at home with his family. He has a tracheostomy and requires a portable respirator, tube feedings, physical and occupational therapy, speech therapy, and special schooling. His mother and father share Jerry's care, assisted by the paternal grandparents and the aunt.

PETER

Now thirteen years old, Peter was born with a congenitally deformed leg that required an above-the-knee amputation when he was age nine. His parents had long since mourned the loss of function in the deformed limb and the actual loss of the limb at amputation. They were actively supporting Peter's growth and his first participation in competitive swimming. His mother called to say how proud they were of Peter and how devastated they were by the sight of him standing on his one leg, ready to dive into the pool with his teammates. They were both surprised and distressed by the reemergence of sadness and hurt, feelings they had put away long ago.

I have borrowed the term "chronic sorrow" from Olshansky (1962) to describe this phenomenon and redefined it in this way: Chronic sorrow is the pervasive sadness experienced over a lifetime by a family with a chronically ill or defective child. This sorrow is experienced most acutely at the time of diagnosis of the child's illness in response to losing a healthy child; it is rekindled with each exacerbation of the disease, at each new developmental phase, and at other unexpected moments. Chronic sorrow is present to some degree in all families with chronically ill children — that is, it is a normal response. The way that a family deals with its chronic sorrow directly influences the family's adaptation and, in turn, the child's response to chronic illness.

Caregivers have identified many factors in the child, the family, the disease and its treatment, and the health care delivery system that contribute to adaptation or maladaptation of chronically ill children and their families; the professional literature is full of references. However, one extremely powerful factor that has been given relatively little attention is chronic sorrow.

REVIEW OF THE LITERATURE

The psychiatric literature describing the mourning that occurs at diagnosis hints at the lifelong process of the grieving. Drotar et al. (1975) reported the results of interviews with the parents of twenty children with congenital malformations. The authors described a hypothetical sequence of parental reactions to the child's birth and focused on the process of attachment. They described mourning as a sequence of reactions: shock; denial; sadness, anger, and anxiety; adaptation; and reorganization. They pointed out that this process of mourning differs from the mourning that follows the death of a child because the congenitally malformed or chronically ill child's life continues and the demands for parental care are great.

Solnit and Stark (1961) noted that the psychological preparation for a new child during pregnancy normally involves the wish for a perfect child and the fear of having a damaged one. It is likely that there is always some discrepancy between the parents' expectations and wishes and their actual newborn. Working out this discrepancy becomes one of the developmental tasks of parenthood that leads to the establishment of healthy family relationships. However, where the discrepancy is too great, as it is with the birth of an ill or defective child or when the parents' wishes are too unrealistic, the work of resolution is difficult and problems may occur. Parents' reactions to their ill or defective child are shaped significantly by the nature and degree of the insult as well as by their other life experiences. Mothers feel particular helplessness and experience a keen sense of failure. Coping with the outer reality of a child with a severe illness or congenital defect and the inner reality of feeling the loss of a desired, normal child requires a great deal of emotional work — work described as mourning.

Tarnow and Tomlinson (1978) described a similar mourning process that occurs in the family of a healthy child when a diagnosis of chronic or long-term disease is made at any time during childhood or adolescence. Parents must readjust their perceptions of an intact and completely healthy child as well as their own immediate and long-term hopes in order to be supportive of the child's adaptation. They must, as well deal with their own guilt (particularly if the disease is inherited or genetically linked) if they are to be capable of responding in a way that is helpful to the child.

Mattson (1972) noted that parents of children with serious, long-term illness mourn the loss of their desired normal child and experience the emergence of feelings of self-blame in regard to the ailing child. When parents become aware of these feelings and can express them, they are better able to accept the reality of the child's disability and its impact on the whole family. A crucial factor in parents' acceptance is their ability to master self-accusatory feelings about having transmitted or in some way caused their child's disorder.

APPLICATION TO CLINICAL PRACTICE

I believe that it is our responsibility as caregivers to recognize the grieving process and the presence of chronic sorrow, to make periodic assessments of how the families of chronically ill children are living and functioning with this sorrow, and to intervene in well-timed, appropriate ways. An ideal time for the initial assessment of family functioning and for therapeutic intervention is at the time of crisis — that is, at the birth of an infant with a congenital malformation or illness or when a child is diagnosed as having a chronic, life-threatening disease. The assessment should include:

1. A thorough family history with special attention to relationships, communication patterns, support networks, recent or significant family losses, ways of coping, and experiences with illness and attitudes toward it.
2. An understanding of the place and role the child occupies in that family system. With a newborn, it is important to know the parents' wishes, expectations, dreams, and hopes for the child. With an older child, it is important to know his or her actual place, as well as parental expectations of what the child might become.

Leahey and Wright (1985) have proposed several types of family intervention. These direct interventions, focused on the cognitive, affective, and behavioral levels of functioning, are especially useful at the time of diagnosis.

1. *Cognitive interventions* include providing information about the illness, suggesting responses the family might have to the child's illness (for example, the impact on marital relations and siblings), offering information about community resources, and providing help with decision making.
2. *Affective interventions* are designed to modify the intense emotions blocking a family's problem-solving efforts. They provide validation of family members' strong feelings of denial, intense anger, guilt, and sadness, sorrow, and resignation or depression.
3. *Behavioral interventions* include encouraging families not to make major adjustments in their lives and encouraging them to seek opportunities for respite.

Updated assessments and interventions over the course of the child's illness are needed as changes occur in the child's medical and developmental status and as major changes occur within the family. Suggested long-term interventions include short-term therapy (counseling) for the family or its individual members, ongoing consultation, group work with parent support groups, and ongoing counseling with the child and family during developmental crisis periods.

Wise and responsible caregivers will recognize that chronic sorrow is an unmeasured but real force in families of chronically ill children, a force that directly influences the development and adaptation of those children over a lifetime. Having done so, they will provide ongoing help for patients and their families as they deal with this problem.

REFERENCES

Drotar, D., A. Baskiewics, N. Irvin, J. Kannel, and M. Klaus. 1975. "The Adaptation of Parents to the Birth of an Infant with a Congenital Malformation: A Hypothetical Model." *Pediatrics* 56:710-717.

Leahey, M. and L. M. Wright. 1985. "Intervening with Families and Chronic Illness." *Family Systems Medicine* 3:60-69.

Mattson, A. 1972. "Long-Term Physical Illness in Childhood: A Challenge to Psychosocial Adaptation." *Pediatrics* 50:801-806.

Olshansky, S. 1962. "Chronic Sorrow: A Response to Having a Mentally Defective Child." *Social Casework* 43:191-192.

Solnit, A. J. and M. H. Stark. 1961. "Mourning the Birth of a Defective Child." *The Psychoanalytic Study of the Child* 16:523-537.

Tarnow, J. D. and N. Tomlinson. 1978. "Juvenile Diabetes Mellitus: Impact on Child and Family." *Psychosomatics* 19:487-491.

The Impact of the Disabled Child on the Family

Sarah Sheets Cook

In order to discuss the impact of a disabled child on the family, we must first define some terms and frames of reference. By *family*, we mean a network of individuals whose personal relationships with each other are characterized by a continuous interchange and by reciprocal causal effects (Miller, cited in Shapiro 1983). Traditionally, family members are consanguineous, but they need not be. A family is viewed as a dynamic system with a complex series of feedback loops in which responsibility for function or dysfunction is distributed among the members. Family systems are open, complex, self-regulating, and capable of transformation.

Within a family, the disabled child is seen as the *identified client*. In some families, *illness* is characterized by clusters of simultaneously occurring symptoms in several members, including the identified client; in other families only the identified client becomes and is seen as being ill (Kellner, cited in Shapiro 1983).

Illness and *disability* are considered synonymous, although objectively they may not be. Each family system is much more than a collection of its constituents: each has its own family mythology passed on from generation to generation, based on fact and fiction, having to do with attitudes toward birth, growth, illness, roles, and death — all of which shape and are shaped by serious disability in a child (Illingsworth et al., cited in Shapiro 1983; Sabbeth 1984).

The impact of a disabled child on a family may be viewed in several different ways. We will discuss this impact from the point

---

Sarah Sheets Cook, RN, MEd, is Assistant Professor of Clinical Nursing and Chairperson, Division of Maternal Child Health Nursing, Columbia University, New York, NY.

© 1988 by The Haworth Press, Inc. All rights reserved.

of view of the child, that of the primary caretakers (parents and siblings), and, finally, from the perspective of the family as a unit.

Since the disabled child is the identified client and the source of numerous stimuli to family responses to his or her illness, it is important to consider briefly the effects of disability on the child. Perrin and Gerrit (1984) have highlighted age of onset as a primary factor influencing the developmental response of the child to his or her disability, in addition to more general factors, including the specific diagnosis; individual differences in temperament and personality; family functioning; social support network; finances; sibling and peer responses; and the responses of teachers, physicians, nurses, and other professionals.

Disability in infants interrupts the consistency and dependability of the family environment. Altered feelings and social responses do not provide the usual positive reinforcement for parenting behaviors. The infants' lack of cognitive awareness of their problems means that they respond only to repeated separations from caretakers, painful experiences, and uncomfortable physical restrictions. The disabled infant's general perception is of a physical and social environment that is nonreinforcing, frightening, and inconsistent.

For toddlers, disability brings unusual restrictions and demands. Repeated episodes of pain, enforced passivity, immobility, separation, and loss of control over procedures, desires, and even diet leads to feelings of defeat, apathy, increased passivity, and clinging. Development of a sense of autonomy and independence is difficult, as is integration of cognition and neuromuscular maturation. Toddlers understand disability only as it affects them and interferes with their activity and choices. In addition, young children's notion that thought has magical power causes them to think that they themselves caused their disability.

Preschoolers who are dealing with disability experience decreased opportunities for peer interaction and peer approval and a diminished sense of initiative and mastery. They tend to have a poor self-image and to be fearful, excessively dependent on adults, and overly sensitive to criticism. Preschoolers' responses to disability are further complicated by their anthropomorphic and simplistic ideas about how the body works and by their cognitive inability to understand the complexity of causative factors or requirements for "recovery."

School-age children worry about their differentness and the interference of disability with peer group activities. School is where the developmental work of this group normally occurs. For a child not to be in school is devastating and leads to problems in developing a sense of self-competence and confidence.

Adolescents with disability must face increased dependence at a time when increased independence is essential. Alterations in body image, which is precarious enough even in average adolescents, create multiple problems that may lead to the feeling of being unattractive and imperfect, isolation and withdrawal, difficulty in establishing meaningful relationships outside the family, and either refusal to comply with medical regimens or the sabotage of them.

A common theme in all developmental stages for children with a disability or chronic illness is stress. Generally speaking, stress, regardless of its source, has a cumulative effect. Factors that mediate or protect the child from this effect include "favorable" home environment, self-esteem, the availability of environmental options, structure and control in the family, and stable relationships with adults (Rutter, cited in Shapiro 1983). The probability of assuring that these criteria exist in the disabled child's world is tenuous at best.

A child's disability can have an impact on the primary caretakers (parents and siblings) in many spheres: financial, social, somatic, behavioral, and conscious or unconscious mental life. It must be remembered, too, that regardless of sphere of influence, the term *impact* has both positive and negative implications. Sabbeth (1984) pointed out that most of the literature about the impact of childhood disability on family focuses on the mother. This raises certain assumptions that may or may not be valid—that a disabled child is more of an insult to the mother than to the father; that mothers are most affected by or have more knowledge about the disability because they are most closely involved with the day-to-day care of the child; that mothers are most influential with children; and that mothers are at home more and are more available for research.

Solnit and Stark (cited in Sabbeth 1984) described a task that seems most relevant to mothers. It involves mourning (whether at birth or later in the child's life) for the loss of the wished-for perfect child and coming to terms with and accepting the child that is. Stage theory is a popular way to conceptualize this process and has been articulated by numerous authors after the Kubler-Ross paradigm — a period of shock, disbelief, and denial; anger, guilt, and resentment; bargaining; depression; and finally, it is hoped, acceptance or reconstruction.

Definitions of *acceptance* are complex and may involve fluctuations in levels or regression to previous stages. Periods of resentment and irritation at the burdens — psychological, physical, and financial — are common. Mothers may develop unrealistically low expectations for the child in order to protect themselves from disappointment (Strand, cited in Shapiro 1983). More common seem to be feelings of anxiety and uncertainty, leading to overprotectiveness and overindulgence toward the child. Depression, unresolved grief, chronic sorrow, or anticipatory mourning are all possible. It should be noted, however, that many of the studies that have produced these conclusions lacked controls and used less-than-rigorous research methodology (Sabbeth 1984).

Less attention has been given to the impact of child disability on fathers. Some studies have indicated long-term personality changes, but none of these studies is conclusive (Sabbeth 1984). There is great variability in fathers' involvement and participation in the care of their disabled children. Traditionally, fathers spend many hours at work, leaving wives and children at home. This absence may foster not only emotional withdrawal, but also avoidance of intense anger, disappointment, and sorrow. A father's sense of helplessness may be exacerbated by the fact that many men are accustomed to working actively to achieve positive results and may be undone by their lack of control over their child's disability or illness. Further, societal stereotypes frequently prohibit men from expressing their feelings or demonstrating vulnerability, and this may increase their sense of isolation.

Marital dysfunction is often mentioned as an effect of a child's disability on both father and mother, even to the point of destroying the relationship. However, it is not clear that a significantly higher divorce rate is characteristic of such families (Shapiro 1983; Sabbeth 1984).

Parents are often extremely concerned about the effect of a child's disability on their other children. A good deal of meaningful, although not necessarily statistically valid material, has been written by parents themselves (Sabbeth 1984). Siblings have described feeling embarrassed about their disabled brother or sister and then feeling guilty about it. They may fear catching the disability or disease. They may envy the extra attention accorded their sibling. They may resent the burdens, real or imagined, of helping to care for the disabled sibling, or fear that they will inherit those burdens when their parents can no longer care for the disabled child. Some are torn between loyalty to home and the disabled sibling and a desire to be out in the normal world and rid of the stigma. Some studies have indicated that siblings are at risk of developing psychosocial problems, especially in school. These problems can include underachievement, lack of friends, fighting, mentation difficulties, and delinquency (Sabbeth 1984). Their own age, sex, and ordinal position, and the severity of their sibling's disability, have been identified as contributing factors in children's responses.

Although members of the health care team are not actual members of the family, physicians especially influence family interaction and response. Physicians are seen as powerful, imbued with magical abilities to "cure" the child if they so wish. Families overtly or covertly attempt to "do everything right" — to adjust appropriately and not to ask too many questions — so that the physicians will think well of them. Similarly, physicians protect themselves against feeling overwhelmed by the pain and helplessness of their patients and families. They may not always have the time, inclination, or training to understand the true impact of the child's disability on the family (Sabbeth 1984).

Families, as units, evolve coping responses, including actions, thoughts, verbalizations, or feelings, which are elicited by the stressors of the disability. One coping response might be the cancellation of all family holidays because the financial drain of the disability is too great or forces the reordering of family priorities and the reallocation of family roles. The family also has a collection of coping resources that are aspects of the external or internal environment and that are not directly or completely under the family's control. Internal coping resources might be a history of family cohesiveness and a success in dealing with previous problems. External coping resources might include formal or informal support systems.

In analyzing the impact of a child's disability on the family as a unit, some assessment of both coping responses and coping resources needs to be made. Successful coping includes meeting such criteria as minimal disruptions of usual family functioning with enforcement of only realistic and necessary restrictions on the disabled child; open, good communication and support among family members; adequate financial resources; and availability and functioning of external support systems. Maladaptive coping includes such phenomena as severe or unchanging denial of the reality of the disability; isolation of the affected child from the rest of the family; hypochondriasis in other family members; projection of angry feelings onto other family members; extreme regression of siblings; rigidity in family system functioning; and unremitting hostility to health care personnel (Shapiro 1983).

Family coping responses can be categorized in ways other than successful or unsuccessful: for example, a purposeful response to an identified stressor may be more effective, regardless of the nature of that response, than randomly chosen or accidental responses. The family that consciously decides to deny their fears about a disabled child in order to continue to support the child in independent functioning may be quite healthy, even though persistent denial is usually seen as maladaptive.

Functionality is another criterion for assessing family coping responses. Any strategy that increases emotional and physical well-being in the family and that maintains its function can be seen as useful and appropriate. The family's perception of their functionality is extremely important here, as is the concept of relating different coping responses and strategies to different stages of the illness or disability process. If the child's disability is one that will result in an earlier-than-expected death, then what is appropriate to coping early in the disability may be inappropriate at the time of the child's death.

There are many unanswered questions regarding the impact of a child's disability on the family as a unit. One of the most intriguing is why, when confronted by equally stressful situations, similar families respond in different ways, one being able to cope better than the other. Another question concerns the identification and management of the psychosomatogenic family — the one whose response to the child's disability exacerbates the problems.

Perrin and Ireys (1984) have discussed the practical aspects of care management of a disabled or chronically ill child that affect family functioning. Comprehensive, individualized health care is often not available in one place from a single group of health care providers. Families experience much stress in trying to coordinate appointments and in getting to them, not to mention paying for them. If the disabled child's diagnosis is rare, available health care providers may not be aware of treatment and management options. Further, if travel and lodging are necessary for medical appointments, the costs are not currently tax deductible.

Families whose child's disability requires a high level of continuous care often "wear out." Their informal support services do not meet their needs or a network of such services is not available to them. They have a great need for respite care — someone who is trustworthy and competent in caring for the disabled child so that the parents can have worry-free time away from the child. Often such care is not available or, if it is, it is not reimbursable by third-party payment.

In general, health care providers and third-party payment groups are not sufficiently aware of the high cost of chronic illness — not only the medical cost but also the cost of time lost from work for direct child care or keeping appointments; the costs of transportation, lodging, telephone, and special supplies; and the emotional cost, which is hard to quantify. Butler (cited in Perrin and Ireys 1984) has noted that the inability to obtain needed services such as family counseling, mental health services, structural modifications to the home, respite care, and homemaker services may ultimately increase the cost of care incurred by both the family and society because the lack of such services leads to inappropriate, episodic care and unnecessary hospitalization and institutionalization.

In summary, we have seen that the impact of the disabled child on the family is extremely complex, involving multiple factors that influence the disabled child, the individual family members, and the family as a unit. Shapiro pointed out (1983:1926) that:

What is still needed is additional research and clinical investigation to clarify concepts such as "family" coping, "adaptive and dysfunctional coping," and to tie these to specific behavioral and cognitive skills which the [health care provider] can integrate into . . . practice.

REFERENCES

Perrin, J. and P. Gerrit. 1984. "Development of Children with Chronic Illness." *Pediatric Clinics of North America* 31(1):19-33.

Perrin, J. and H. Ireys. 1984. "Services for Chronically Ill Children and Their Families." *Pediatric Clinics of North America* 31(1):235-251.

Sabbeth, B. 1984. "Understanding the Impact of Chronic Childhood Illness on Families." *Pediatric Clinics of North America* 31(1):47-57.

Shapiro, J. 1983. "Family Reactions and Coping Strategies in Response to the Physically Ill or Handicapped Child: A Review." *Social Science Medicine* 17(1):913-931.

BIBLIOGRAPHY

Beckman, P. J. 1983. "Influence of Child Characteristics on Stress in Families with Handicapped Infants." *American Journal of Mental Deficiency* 88(2): 150-156.

Buschman, P. et al. 1985. "Anger in the Clinical Setting." *American Journal of Maternal Child Nursing* 10(5):313-337.

Crnic, K. A. et al. 1983. "Adaptation in the Family with a Mentally Retarded Child." *American Journal of Mental Deficiency* 88(2):125-138.

Ferrari, M. 1984. "Chronic Illness: Psychosocial Effects on Siblings." *Journal of Child Psychology and Psychiatry* 25(3):459-476.

Frey, J. 1984. "Family Systems Approach to Illness Maintaining Behaviors in Chronically Ill Adolescents." *Family Process* 23(2):251-260.

Hobbs, J., J. Perrin, and H. Ireys. 1985. *Chronically Ill Children and Their Families*. San Francisco: Jossey-Bass.

Racy, J. 1983. "Families and Chronic Disease." *Arizona Medicine* 40(12): 854-885.

Some Aspects of Psychosocial Sequelae to Treatment of Scoliosis in Adolescent Girls

Frances K. Forstenzer
David Price Roye, Jr.

This article is based on the preliminary results of our study of the psychosocial sequelae of scoliosis in adolescents. This longitudinal study, using the Forstenzer-Roye Questionnaire for Assessment of Adolescent Girls with Scoliosis (copyright 1984), is in progress and will continue over an extended time. This study was undertaken because concern for this population was expressed by parents, teachers, mental health professionals, physicians, and nurses, mainly with regard to the chronicity of the diagnosis and the sensitive age at which the condition is usually identified.

RESPONSES TO DIAGNOSIS

The diagnosis of scoliosis in girls is made primarily at the beginning of adolescence. This is a particularly vulnerable period in terms of the development of a girl's self-image in relation to self-esteem. A multitude of physical changes usually take place at this time, as well as the beginning of sexual development. At this age, girls focus great emotional and mental energy on concerns about

Frances K. Forstenzer, LCSW, is affiliated with the Center for Living, Baltimore, MD. David Price Roye, Jr., MD, is Assistant Professor of Orthopedic Surgery, College of Physicians and Surgeons, Columbia University, New York, NY.

© 1988 by The Haworth Press, Inc. All rights reserved.

their weight, shape, hair, skin, and total appearance. Acute, almost painful self-consciousness is common. The adolescent is not only vulnerable to self-criticism but also to the scrutiny of her peers. Members of the peer group study each other carefully in an effort to understand the norms so that each can struggle to look like the others at the same time that she tries to find an individual identity.

Scoliosis, like any other chronic condition, has long-term implications for the patient's sense of self. She will have to deal with issues of loss on both an immediate and an ongoing basis, and will understand and integrate these issues in accordance with her developmental level, personality, and home situation, as well as the responses of her parents.

The latency-age child enters adolescence with concerns and worries about the changes beginning in her body. In addition, she brings with her the fantasy of the beautiful and perfect woman she can become "when I grow up." Although the word *perfect* means different things to different young girls, the fantasy is precious to them. Their visions of possible adult roles are generally peopled with images of the imagined "perfect" adults they might become.

The degree to which physical "perfection" is psychologically valued depends not only on the images of society as a whole but also on family values and the health or pathology of the parents in their relationship to the child. For example, a beginning adolescent who feels appreciated, valued, and "pretty" in the eyes of her father will have an easier time adjusting her self-image and her sense of self than a girl whose father frequently criticizes her appearance, as in "Comb your hair," "Change your clothes," or "It's too bad you're not pretty like. . . ." Similarly, a girl whose mother is heavily invested in the perfection of her house, herself, her life, and her children will find an imperfect child seriously threatening in several areas at once.

The adolescent who is dealing with a diagnosis of scoliosis must cope with loss of the fantasy of the perfect adult that she imagined she might one day become. Whatever else will happen to her in terms of her self-image, she will have to integrate this fact about her body into her sense of who she is now and who she will be forever. Although no girl, even without scoliosis, can grow into adulthood without giving up this fantasy of the perfect self, the addition of a specific condition that requires medical attention (as opposed to "My nose is too big" or "My hair is too curly") can have a strongly deflating emotional effect. The acceptance of a chronic medical condition is a strong dose of reality.

As with any other trauma, the child will deal with the loss of this fantasy by depending on her core sense of self. If that self is fragile and easily fragmented, it will be more difficult for her to absorb the concept of a chronic diagnosis that is usually perceived as an attack on the self, requiring psychological reorganization. In addition to responses related to a core self, the child will respond out of her individual personality traits, such as anxiety, fearfulness, and cognitive and processing abilities.

In addition to the loss that the child will sustain, the parents will lose the "perfect" and totally "well" child they may have had before the diagnosis. If the child has had other medical problems, the parents may perceive the scoliosis as one more imperfection that further validates the sense of the child's inadequacy. If the child has not had previous medical problems, the scoliosis may become the focus of the now "not perfect" child.

Parents with strong, well-functioning egos are able to absorb this loss, reorganize their concept of the child, and respond appropriately in the parental roles of reality testing, support, exploration, comfort, and assessment of priorities. More fragile parents, particularly those with narcissistic or hysterical personality disorders, will react as if they have been attacked and have lost some valued piece of themselves. Their ability to parent effectively will be compromised, and they may experience periods of uncontrollable narcissistic rage or wild hysterical behavior. The child whose parents respond in this way will have to deal with the loss of unconditional positive regard and the withdrawal of a certain amount of affection, as well as the loss of her own fantasies and self-concepts. Thus, the child will be attempting to find an adaptive pattern at a time when she has less available parenting to draw on. Mourning for both of these losses may be more than the child can handle at the same time without other emotional support.

TREATMENT

Scoliosis is usually treated by three different modalities: (1) monitoring over time, (2) bracing, and (3) surgery. Each of these modalities has numerous inherent difficulties for the child.

Monitoring — that is, seeing the patient every four to six months and checking the progress of the curvature by radiography — is certainly the most benign form of treatment. Between visits, the child leads an ordinary life and does not have to relate to the scoliosis at all. Interestingly, however, it has become obvious through interviews with these children that monitoring creates tremendous anxiety and pressure each time the need for further treatment is evaluated. Some of the girls report not sleeping the night before, shaking with fright, and not wanting to look at the radiographs. "I knew it had gotten worse, I just knew it!" said one fourteen-year-old. When she was told for the second or third time that it was only a little worse and still did not require further treatment, she replied, "It will get worse, you'll see. It will keep getting worse. Nothing good ever happens to me!"

Parents also respond to monitoring with anxiety, particularly when the diagnosis of scoliosis has special meaning to them in terms of narcissistic injury. One mother, whose daughter had an eight-degree curvature that had remained the same over many visits, said, "Look at her shoulder — it's a little higher than the other one. It must be getting worse. It shows so much in some clothes. I see some girls in braces here and I don't know how the parents can stand it!" This was said in the waiting room and was audible not only to her daughter but to several other families as well. As a result of this mother's anxiety and her need to see her daughter as a "perfect" extension of herself, she was unable to feel or respond to the child's anxieties and fears, creating an empathic failure of considerable magnitude. Such failures, repeated over time, have a significant influence on the child's personality development.

Needless to say, bracing is also a considerable emotional burden for the child to carry. Unlike monitoring, bracing is pervasive, since the child initially must wear the brace for twenty-three hours a day. Although low-profile braces are not as visible as the old Milwaukee brace, the child must still concern herself with every article of clothing ("Will it fit?" "Does it go under or over the brace?" "Do I need a bigger size?" "Will I look fatter?") for an indefinite period that may extend through her entire adolescence. In addition to the issues related to clothing and appearance, the adolescent girl who is dealing with her newly emerging sexuality has the additional burden of how to hug or touch, since she is in a situation of "If you hug me, you hug my brace." The interpersonal issues surface in terms of changing and dressing in front of other girls as well as in relation to boys.

The child who must wear a brace also faces continuous monitoring of the curvature and the attendant anxiety of decisions about whether or not the brace is proving effective, whether or not the hours she must wear it can be shortened, when and if she can stop wearing the brace, and, finally, if the brace is not effective, whether or not surgery is required. Each visit to the physician becomes a serious event during which an important decision may be made. Each time a new treatment plan evolves, the child has to assimilate a slightly different concept of herself and, once again, must face the need to relinquish old fantasies. If most of these occasions are handled with a high degree of empathy, the child may actually develop a strong, resilient sense of self that can be carried over to other situations. On the other hand, all of the issues related to bracing are emotionally weighted for both parents and child, and many opportunities arise for their response levels to be less than optimal, making it likely that the child's self-esteem will then be damaged.

Surgery is certainly the most radical approach to the treatment of scoliosis. This is serious surgery, with all the sequelae of anesthesia, as well as those of the surgery itself. The child's body is changed forever: Harrington rods stay where they are put, and there is a long scar down the girl's back.

The psychological issues associated with serious surgery are manifold: fear of pain, death, physician error, separation, hospitalization, and being incapacitated come to mind immediately. In addition, an adolescent must deal with the temporary renewal of dependence after having achieved a degree of independence. And, since we are describing female patients who are primarily treated by male physicians, the issue of sexual invasion must also be considered.

It is interesting to note that what may be considered medically radical may in fact be psychologically conservative. Girls who are treated surgically for scoliosis are braced for six months after surgery and then followed yearly. Thus, for surgical patients, the length of time that they must be encumbered by a brace and be anxious while the curvature is being followed is far shorter than for other patients. Because the length of postoperative bracing is limited, every aspect of adolescent development is not affected.

So far, there is no clear evidence to indicate which approach represents the greatest sense of loss for the child. And, in any event, it seems unlikely that medical decisions will be based on psychological considerations. However, if more research can be done in this area, the question of the flavor and feel of patients' entire adolescent experience can someday become part of the decision-making process. Although more knowledge is needed in this area, it seems clear that in order for the adolescent patient to emerge with as little psychological damage as possible, it is desirable for the treatment team to be sensitive and responsive to psychosocial issues.

BIBLIOGRAPHY

Anderson, B. 1979. "Carole, A Girl Treated with Bracing." *American Journal of Nursing* 152 (Sept.):1598.

Clayson, D. and D. Levine. 1976. "Adolescent Scoliosis Patients—Personality Patterns and Effects of Corrective Surgery." *Clinical Orthopedics* 116 (May):919-1002.

Clayson, D., D. Levine, and B. Mahon. 1981. "Pre-Op Personality Characteristics as Predictors of Post-Op Physical and Psychological Patterns in Scoliosis." *Spine* 691 (1):9-12.

IV. DEALING WITH
LIFE-THREATENING DISEASE

Care of the Dying Adolescent
and the Bereaved Family

Barbara B. Johansen

Each individual in the family responds to the diagnosis of an adolescent's terminal illness in a way that is consistent with his or her own personality structure, past experience, current crises, and the particular meaning or special circumstances associated with the threatened loss. To obtain the most positive results, medical professionals should address the complete family system.

Ultimately, when a child is diagnosed with a terminal disease, the entire family is the patient. Roles within the family are altered. Parents' ability to handle day-to-day problems often declines. What they need is a listener who is willing to tell them that what they are experiencing in terms of their lack of zest for life, indecision, and feeling overwhelmed by the simple tasks of daily living are normal responses. Anxiety can be relieved by knowing that being frightened and distracted is normal and that being depressed is common.

Barbara B. Johansen is Family Education Specialist and President, Change of Pace Experiences, Inc., New Canaan, CT.

© 1988 by The Haworth Press, Inc. All rights reserved.

STRESSES FACED BY THE FAMILY

These stresses include intellectual problems and pragmatic tasks as well as social, emotional, and spiritual challenges. They can be dealt with as a series of positive tasks or challenges — as opportunities for learning, positive growth, and renewed faith and meaning for a better life. Personally, my family accepted Paul's diagnosis as a challenge to make it the most positive experience we could. We had gone through the lingering cancer deaths of both my parents and had a positive role model in each of them. We also had two close friends whose children had cancer that was in remission. We saw how their relationships were strained and communication became a problem.

COMMUNICATION

Relationships characterized by warmth, respect, and mutual trust among the medical care team, the family, and the adolescent patient are extremely beneficial. Communication that is open, honest, and intimate enough to allow for disagreements without jeopardizing the relationship is vitally important in this stress-filled atmosphere. Genuine concern for the family's nonmedical as well as medical needs is extremely important to the support of the family and the well-being of the patient.

Parents must be good to themselves and all the family. I urge parents not to overindulge the patient. The effects can be disastrous: a demanding, spoiled, unlikeable patient, a negative response from the medical staff, and problems for the other children and family members.

ADOLESCENTS' NEEDS

Young people's needs do not change when diagnosis and loss of faculties occur. They still need to be with and be accepted by their peers. I have heard over and over again from teenage patients, "I am still me—I haven't changed inside my head and my feelings just because of a diagnosis, chemo, or radiation." After diagnosis, young people, in fact, often put themselves on an accelerated track for experiencing life—denial can be part of this race with time.

Parents are prone to worry more than the child. It is important to build open communication systems and a team approach to care that involves the patient, the family, and the medical staff. Information should be structured carefully, and instructions should be given in ways that help the patient understand their advantage. Medical personnel as well as other caregivers often see adolescent patients and their families as passive recipients in a vertical process. Understanding that they can take care of their bodies and minds is important for these patients. Offering them methods of achieving this, such as imagery and relaxation techniques, is helpful. Medical personnel and other caregivers should encourage adolescent patients in their new awareness. For catastrophically ill adolescents, tuning in to their bodies and responding to their bodies' messages and rhythms can be a powerful tool to help them create feelings of well-being.

Having someone to talk with is vital. It is to be expected that adolescents will resent the sick role, and knowing this can relieve anxious minds. The patients should be encouraged to ask questions, and their questions should be answered honestly. Building trust with adolescents is particularly important—they hold truth high in esteem and can usually read through the blurred statements sent their way.

In helping the patient, one should offer unconditional love, avoiding criticism or value judgments. Caregivers should keep a sense of humor and use it—the patient has one that also needs exercise. Parents and staff should endeavor to examine, understand, and cope with their own feelings so that they can become more effective listeners. Conversation on subjects that interest the teenager should be encouraged and the illness should be seen from the teenager's point of view. To improve communication with the patient, it is necessary to avoid medical jargon, find out the patient's expectations, and identify the patient's anxieties.

FAMILY, SCHOOL, AND COMMUNITY

Informal involvements with the family by the school, community, and church are significant links to the successful wholistic care of the terminally ill adolescent patient. It is imperative to maintain and build these links from the time of diagnosis. Patients and their parents should be encouraged to allow their community to love them — to call out for help from friends and neighbors and see it as an opportunity for others to feel good about themselves. Others often feel helpless and impotent, but they can be helped to approach the situation creatively. Frequently, assuring the siblings that they, too, are important can be done best by a close friend of the family or by a neighbor who will share time with the siblings and do things that the children enjoy.

It is helpful to all involved to include the school nurse, as well as the patients' individual teachers and staff, having one concerned faculty member and student serve as liaisons for communication. I know that the open, supportive systems of active involvement elected by many of the school personnel had a strongly positive impact on my son's wellness and his attendance at school. I believe that the enthusiastic cooperation of his doctors and nurses was most helpful in facilitating this response.

When the student attends school irregularly or not at all, it is vital that contact with peers be maintained. One way of helping to achieve this is a two-way communication system that uses the telephone lines and consists of small boxes, one placed in the patients' room and the other in the classroom. The system is operated by a pressure-sensitive button or switch. Again, I call on our personal experience: when we used this system, visible vitality came into Paul's body as he heard his classes called to order. He could answer or be questioned when his energies were up. He continued to be an integral part of his classes, and his friends would stop by on breaks to chat, tell jokes, or relate that day's "hot news." This means of teaching is often discouraged by educational systems — they prefer to send in a tutor on schedule. Because both methods of instruction are not offered, a choice must be made, but the family should be made aware of the options. In light of the prognosis, it is important to measure which method offers the richer quality of life for the terminally ill adolescent.

Medical professionals are role models and have a unique opportunity to encourage young people to do informative projects on their disease for school reports. I have seen this occur with dynamic effects for all concerned.

TEEN SUPPORT PROGRAMS

I emphasize the need to establish support programs within hospitals for the interaction of inpatient and outpatient adolescents. Supportive interaction gives renewed purpose to their lives. Informal rap programs built around snacks, fun foods, and their kind of music work well. "Come and bring a friend" meetings usually have good results, although sometimes the concept is slow in getting started with teenagers. Usually the patient and friends leave such sessions with new perspectives and deeper understanding of each other. Offering them phone and address lists of those attending is important to continuing the support network. The phone works wonders. As one teenager said about his phone pal, "When I'm helping others, I forget about my own situation and feel lots better when I'm through." It is important for the adolescent patient to live each moment as alive as possible rather than to adapt to the death process. Feeling helpful to others fosters this.

PARENT SUPPORT GROUPS

In the community, the family is isolated in their experience. Through a mutual support group, they are less vulnerable to that desperate feeling of aloneness. The group also enables them to connect to role models in other parents and to learn about successful methods of survival. Many hospitals have developed effective programs to meet these needs. Getting involved in this type of support community builds the foundation for the support network that can be so uniquely effective as the adolescent patient's condition deteriorates. Candlelighters, a national organization with local chapters, offers parent support opportunities and, on occasion, programs for the patients and their siblings.

Parent Burnout

Parents need to feel affirmed in this desperate situation. Change of Pace Experiences (COPE) is an organization serving the tri-state area of New York, New Jersey, and Connecticut. COPE attempts to help the parents of children who are in treatment to achieve this affirmation by offering them one-day and weekend opportunities, at no cost, to step back from the rigors of daily caregiving into a respite setting for the purpose of finding renewal, revitalization, and reinspiration. Through the experience of these educational and support programs, offered in an elective three-track mode that addresses the needs of mind, spirit, and body, the parents return home better caregivers to their children.

Parents often will not give themselves permission to separate from the patient. COPE, as an adjunct to parents' caregiving and recommended by medical staff treating their child, finds the parents making concerted efforts to participate. The number of parents who return to the program, as well as their introduction of the program to others, indicates both the need for it and its positive effects. Escape is necessary for all of us. Burnout can occur — how can it be prevented? Just as the dying teenager needs to maintain connections with friends in order to "escape," so do the parents need escapes as well. Many find theirs in COPE. Parents listening to other parents offering reassurance does reduce stress and helps them to cope more effectively.

ADOLESCENTS IN THE FINAL STAGES OF LIFE

When adolescents feel less helpless and frustrated, they may, in turn, be more cooperative and reliable patients. In this way they can be helpful to their parents, family, friends, and staff as well, and feel good about themselves in the process.

A personalized room is very important to patients. Moving them to a new location for their last days should be given much serious consideration — quality of life, not quantity, should be examined. Building on the honest, open communication systems established earlier often enables patients to make the best recommendations for this time in their lives.

Most adolescents want to be reassured that their friends will not forget them, and very often they want to write a will. This is an important piece of business and can often be directly or indirectly implemented by the medical staff.

Informing visitors of the patient's condition is very important. Medical staff are often unaware of how disconcerting the changed appearance of the patient is to those who do not visit daily. I usually tried to have a variety of cookies and juice available as a distraction so that visitors could focus on them until they felt more at ease.

Encouraging brothers and sisters to offer their help gives them a feeling of importance and diminishes any feelings of neglect. I visited a teenage boy whose mother was exhausted and whose little sister was whining for attention. The mother wanted very much to fall into her chair and visit with me. Then her son gave her a sign that he needed something to eat. She started to cry: "Will I never have a moment to myself?" I could recall the feeling well. I asked her if her little girl enjoyed feeding her brother. She looked shocked and then said, "No, she's too little to help with his care." I turned to the three-year-old girl and asked her if she would try feeding her brother so that her mother and I could visit. A little reluctantly, the mother gave the girl the tiny spoon and cup. I covered the patient with a blanket and a large towel and the little sister took her place. All of us then had our time and the emotional space that we needed and felt good about helping and being helped. The chortles from the boy and his sister clearly indicated their feelings.

DEATH AND BEREAVEMENT

If it seems at all within reason to have the adolescent die at home, I urge that the necessary measures be implemented. The cooperative efforts of the physician and a home care support nursing network are imperative for this to happen effectively. Many community hospice groups do not include pediatric home care programs. Parents can and do learn to step in as primary administrants of powerful drugs when necessary. Allowing parents the opportunity to continue as effective caregivers to their child is a "gift" to both the parents and the child. The parents continue to feel helpful to their child to the end, allowing their love to flow and encouraging them to live each moment.

Preventing the parents from feeling alone or abandoned is of primary importance. Outside support systems must continue to the death of the child and must continue for the parents in the months that follow.

Each family member is unique and will respond to the death of the adolescent child in his or her own way. Learning to respect each other's different forms of grief is important but often difficult. The parents are often confused by each other's responses to their loss. It is often impossible to comfort when one experiences a comparable grief. Communication often becomes blurred in the absence of the patient as a focus. Spouses often have unconscious expectations about their partners' grief responses. When these responses do not occur, serious problems can develop in their relationship. Setting up expectations of others usually spells trouble in relationships. It is important for parents to reach out to each other in this confusing time with affirming, unconditional love.

Medical professionals should stay connected to the family for a reasonable period after the patient's death. In the initial bereavement period, the significant impact of their continued interest in the family, indicated even by a phone call, is a vital help in enabling the family to move on positively with life. When members of the medical team do reach out in this way, it is useful if they invite the parents to share their memories, even the dark ones, and assist them in focusing on their present opportunity to celebrate all living things. Parents face the existential problem of making sense out of a fateful circumstance that does not occur frequently in our experience. They are challenged to examine their faith and spiritual integrity and their perceptions of themselves as victims. Many are reluctant to complete the final acknowledgment of the death and so put off ordering a gravestone, choosing a permanent location for the urn, or making whatever decisions their tradition involves. This hinders them from getting on with life.

The help of a family therapist is often positive throughout the grief experience. Behavior modification and mutual respect can occur more rapidly with outside professional assistance. Within families, new awareness of each other's loss comes to light. Professionals involved in treating the child can direct the family to this type of resource for working out their grief. Too often, I have seen families floundering around in isolation at this point, and I have seen them losing touch with each other. Some medical centers are taking on the responsibility of offering bereavement support programs for the parents. It is important that this caregiving task for the bereaved family be completed by the familiar facility.

Losing a child is desperately difficult. I believe that it is helpful for parents in this situation to focus on their own roots. The process of grieving for a child is relevant to other life loss experiences. It is relevant to examine the family's response to illness, loss, and death, looking at three generations. Parents anticipating the death of their child would be helping themselves if they would talk with each other about how their own parents, grandparents, and relatives responded to loss and death. It can also be useful for parents to explore together how they each coped with other losses during their single lives and how, as a couple, they have responded to losses — the loss of job, moving to a new community, the death of a pet, and so on — during their married lives. Definite patterns of response can be discovered in the midst of this devastating experience; a deeper understanding and more sensitive acceptance of self and spouse can be developed.

As a parent who has lost a child, I know we have a choice: to go on celebrating each moment of life or just to exist and live in our grief and depression. It has not been easy. It is not all black or white — a balance is necessary, and time does help. Being alive in each moment takes effort, and I am not always successful. When I fail, I do make an effort to step back and reassess where I am.

At these times, I usually discover that I am tuned in to my fears of the future or to my sorrows. As Paul lived with the knowledge of his impending death, he taught us the importance of unconditional love and the celebration of each moment of life. Life does continue after diagnosis of a child's terminal illness and even after the child's death, but the quality of one's life is a matter of one's own choice.

Depression, Denial, and Withdrawal in Mothers of Seriously Ill Children and Adolescents

Elizabeth J. Susman
Philip A. Pizzo

The existing literature on the parents of seriously ill children focuses primarily on the grief that follows the death of a child. It is likely, however, that anticipatory grief, the initial phase of the grieving process, begins well before the death of a child and can result in altered parental behavior that has a significant impact on the child. The manifestations of anticipatory grieving are similar to depression, and include sadness, inability to concentrate, and underactivity. These parental behaviors potentially deprive the ill child of a nurturant, empathic, and physically indulgent parent. The emotional or physical absence of the parent may leave the child feeling afraid, lonely, and abandoned.

Indeed, there is growing recognition that parents must acquire a variety of new skills in order to cope with the stress of parenting a seriously ill child. One reason there has been little understanding of the impact of anticipatory grieving on parents is that the parents generally are assigned the demanding role of providing comfort and support to the child. The presence of the parent presumably helps the child cope with the frightening experience of hospitalization and painful medical procedures. Although a parent's nurture is comforting to the child, it may be highly stressful for the parent. Binger et

Elizabeth J. Susman, PhD, is Senior Staff Fellow, National Institute of Mental Health, Bethesda, MD. Philip A. Pizzo is affiliated with the National Institute of Health and is Chief of Pediatrics, Oncology Branch at the National Cancer Institute.

al. (1969) found that 50 percent of the parents of the leukemic children studied reacted so emotionally to the diagnosis that psychiatric help was indicated. However, referral to a psychiatrist might depend on the parent population or the tendency of the primary physician to refer a family to a psychiatrist. Findings from any one study may grossly overestimate or underestimate the severity of the problem. In any case, the demands of providing ongoing supportiveness for a sick child may not allow parents the opportunity to deal with their own feelings of depression, guilt, and anxiety.

Parents may cope with their anticipatory grief either by denial or withdrawal. We addressed the question of whether or not distinct patterns that reflect denial and withdrawal are observable in mothers' interactions with their seriously ill hospitalized children and adolescents. We hypothesized that if denial were the primary method of coping, mothers could be expected to continue to interact with their children throughout the course of the illness. Other mothers might withdraw, which could help to protect them from the intense grief that they might view as imminent. Thus, if withdrawal were the primary method of coping, mothers could be expected to interact less and less with their children as the children became increasingly ill.

SAMPLE AND OBSERVATION OF BEHAVIOR

The patients whose mothers were studied were all children or adolescents who had cancer. These patients had not responded to conventional treatment regimens and subsequently participated in a life-threatening experimental treatment regimen designed to test the efficacy of high doses of chemotherapy agents. The first group of mothers were ones whose children died during or shortly after participating in the treatment regimen (N = 6). The second group consisted of mothers whose children lived months or years beyond the end of the same treatment regimen (N = 9).

The mothers' behavior was observed and coded daily as part of a study on the impact of a life-threatening illness on the social and emotional development of children (Susman et al. 1981). The behavior of the mothers was coded on two dimensions, Role and Behavior. The Role categories assessed were *nonsocial* (not interacting with the child), *initiates an interaction with the child*, and *reciprocates to an initiation by the child*. The Behavior categories were active (watching television or playing games with the child), *vocal* (engaging in extended conversations), *passive* (physically proximal but not interacting with the child), and *physical* (assisting the child with procedures or other activities).

Patterns of Individual Behavior

The first phase of the analysis addressed the behavior of each mother at different points in her child's illness. These single-subject analyses were done (1) to determine whether the mothers of children who died consistently interacted with their children at a low level throughout the treatment period or whether the pattern of their interaction had changed as the child became increasingly ill, and (2) to identify the point in the treatment regimen at which mothers appear at risk for psychological problems.

The clinical status of the child was evaluated by absolute granulocyte counts, referred to hereafter as counts. We have discussed the rationale for using counts as an indicator of clinical status in our previous papers (e.g., Susman et al. 1981). Briefly, counts indicate the degree of chemotherapy toxicity, declining as the toxicity increases. Low counts mean that the child is extremely susceptible to life-threatening infections. Children and parents are aware of this susceptibility and therefore experience a great deal of anxiety when counts are decreasing. During this time the child also experiences the greatest degree of somatic distress—for example, in addition to infections there may be fevers and mucous membrane irritations. To analyze the behavior of mothers at different points in the child's illness, counts were divided into three phases: Phase 1, counts above $500/mm^3$, the initial phase of treatment; Phase 2, counts below $500/mm^3$; and Phase 3, counts above $500/mm^3$, the recovery phase.

The behavior of the six mothers whose children died was compared with the behavior of six randomly chosen mothers from the group whose children survived. The data on three mothers from the group whose children died (mothers 1, 2, and 3) and the data on three mothers from the group whose children survived (mothers 4, 5, and 6) illustrate our findings. Figure 1 shows the relative percent of the four mothers' behaviors across days of treatment and counts per mm^3. Chemotherapy was generally given on day 2 of the observation period. Observations were terminated when patients became too ill to interact with their caregivers.

Mother 1 (mother of an adolescent female) initially engaged in high levels of vocalization with her daughter. After day 2, her vocalizations declined until day 8. This mother did not vocalize or play with her daughter from day 9 through the remaining nine days of observation, with the exception of a moderately high level of play on day 13. After day 8, she was absent for four out of ten days. When she was present, she engaged in either passive or physical caretaking behaviors. In general, the nurturant quality of this mother's behavior declined across days of treatment. She gradually withdrew completely from her child.

Mother 2 (mother of an adolescent male) engaged in a variety of behaviors during the initial phase of treatment, which continued while the boy's counts were low. After day 7, she was absent for five of the six days of observation, with the exception of day 11, when she both exhibited passive behavior and vocalized to her son. As her son became increasingly ill, this mother withdrew from him.

Mother 3 (mother of an early adolescent male) also engaged in a variety of behaviors during the initial phase of treatment. This pattern of interaction continued even while her son's counts were low. An unusual feature of this child's history was that he exhibited many behavior problems, both before treatment (e.g., running away from the hospital) and during treatment (e.g., resisting procedures). He dropped out of the observational study a few days before he died. A second unusual feature of this child's history was that he died within a few days after developing chemotherapy related complications, although when his counts were low and he was quite ill his clinical status had not progressively deteriorated as did that of the majority of patients in the sample. The fact that his death was unanticipated may explain why his mother did not show the pattern of withdrawal typical of the other mothers.

In all, four of the six mothers whose children died interacted with

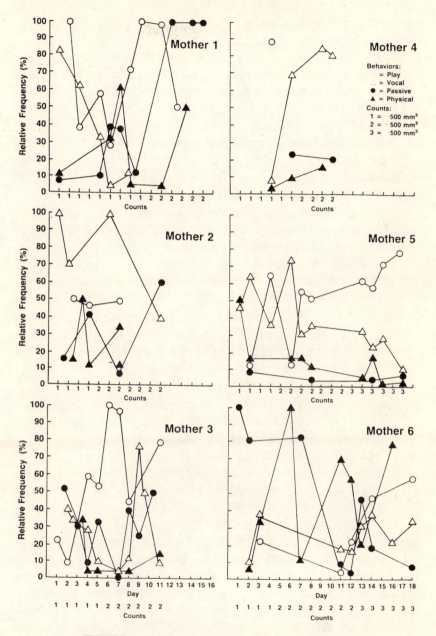

FIGURE 1. Relative Frequency of Mother Behaviors

their children less and less as the children's physical condition deteriorated. However, it is not the mere absence of social interaction that may be traumatic to the ill child. The affective quality of interactions also appeared to decrease as the child's condition worsened. When they did interact, these four mothers tended not to play with or talk to their children, but instead sat passively by the bedside or carried out routine physical activities. What is unknown is whether the behavior patterns observed here reflect the reactions of mothers to their children's deteriorating condition or reactions to stressful situations in general. (Findings from the single-subject analyses are available upon request from the first author.)

The next findings are from three mothers in the group whose children survived. Mother 4 (mother of an adolescent male) was absent during the initial phase of treatment. When her son's counts were low, she vocalized to him. She also engaged in physical and passive behavior during this phase of treatment. This mother withdrew from her son during the recovery phase of his treatment.

Mother 5 (mother of a late adolescent female) interacted with her daughter through a variety of behaviors during the initial phase of treatment. She was absent for four days when her daughter's counts were low. Again, she interacted with her daughter in a variety of ways during the recovery phase of treatment.

Mother 6 (mother of a late adolescent male) exhibited high levels of passive and physical behavior during the initial phase of her son's treatment. She was absent for four days when his counts were low. She interacted with her son through a variety of behaviors during his recovery period. This child was very ill when he began treatment, which may explain her low level of interaction with him during the initial treatment phase.

These three mothers, as well as the others whose children survived, tended to withdraw as their children became increasingly ill—that is, when counts were low—but their withdrawal did not last as long as that of mothers whose children died. Mothers in this group tended to increase interaction with their children during the recovery phase. Furthermore, the mothers in this group tended to exhibit both nurturant and nonnurturant behavior throughout the different phases of illness.

Patterns of Group Behavior

The second phase of the analysis was intended to answer the question of whether or not there were differences in the frequencies of behavior between the two groups of mothers. The data used in the analysis were the mean relative frequency of the Role and Behavior dimension categories collapsed across all days of observation. Chi-square analysis of the Role dimension categories by group (mothers of children who died and mothers of children who survived) revealed a significant association between Role and group, χ^2 $(df = 2) = 8.12, p < .05$. Mothers of the children who died were more likely to be nonsocial and were less likely to initiate an interaction than mothers of the survivors. The two groups did not differ on the *reciprocates an interaction* category. Chi-square analysis of the Behavior dimension categories by group also revealed a significant association between behavior and group, χ^2 $(df = 3) = 15.24, p < .01$. Mothers of the patients who died were less likely to engage in play and vocal behaviors than mothers in the group whose children survived. The two groups were similar in their levels of passive and physical behavior. Thus, different behavior patterns were observed in the two groups of mothers.

Patterns of Coping

Our findings indicate that caring for seriously ill children can have observable effects on the behavior of mothers. Mothers showed distinctly different behavior patterns depending on the outcome of their child's illness. Mothers in both groups tended to withdraw as their children became increasingly ill, but the withdrawal of mothers whose children survived was of shorter duration than that of mothers whose children died.

In the group of mothers whose children died, not only did the quantity of mother-child interaction decline, but the quality of that interaction also declined as their children became increasingly ill. Withdrawal was most pronounced in the nurturant behaviors of vocalization and play. Although mothers of seriously ill children may be physically close to the children, they appear to provide less nurturing and warmth than mothers of less seriously ill children. In general, the behavior pattern observed in the group of mothers whose children died is more indicative of a pattern of withdrawal than a pattern of denial.

With regard to the meaning of withdrawal, two issues should be considered: the sampling procedure used and the relationship between withdrawal and anticipatory grief. Although the mothers of the children who died appeared to withdraw more than the mothers of children who survived, this difference must be interpreted in relation to the sampling procedure. Mother-child interaction was observed until the child either became too ill to interact or recovered and left the hospital. Thus, the findings based on the total days of observation may be biased. If the child became too sick to interact, the observations were discontinued, which may have biased the data toward withdrawal for the group of mothers whose children survived. If the child recovered, mothers tended to increase their interactions as their children's clinical status improved, which may have biased the findings toward nonwithdrawal. Thus, for the group of mothers whose children died, although the overall pattern of behavior indicates withdrawal, that may reflect the reality that their children were sicker and less able to interact. What is unknown is whether or not the observed withdrawal reflects behavior that is typical of mothers' reactions to parenting an ill child.

With respect to the meaning of withdrawal and anticipatory grief, it is important to note that all of the children in the study had failed to respond to conventional treatments. However, most of the parents viewed the experimental treatment as a potential cure, or at least as having the potential to lengthen their child's life. At the point in the treatment regimen when it became clear that a child was terminally ill, the mother may have withdrawn as a method of coping with the child's death. Parents may appropriately grieve over the imminent death of a child. This pattern of coping is different from coping with the possibility that a child who is undergoing therapy may die. Thus, withdrawal can be viewed as an effective parental coping behavior.

Withdrawal from their children may also be emotionally detrimental to both the mothers and their children. As counts go down and children become increasingly ill, mothers may realize the seriousness of the illness. This recognition may precipitate the sadness, underactivity, and inability to concentrate that are characteristic symptoms of depression. The mother's withdrawal from her child may partially shield her from deeply disturbing feelings. It also minimizes contact with awkward situations, such as talking to her child about the future. In addition, although she may not want to be with her child, she also may feel guilty about not wanting to be there. Part of her guilt may be related to a feeling that she has given up prematurely (Goldfogel 1972).

Another reason for withdrawal is that the mother may feel helpless to expedite her child's recovery and in relation to the highly technical medical care that her child requires. At the same time that mothers are feeling helpless, nurses and doctors are often attempting to provide life-saving care to the child. Unfortunately, it is generally difficult for nurses and doctors to provide both medical care to the child and intensive psychological support to mother. Alternative sources of support for mothers require exploration.

A mother's withdrawal may have many emotionally deleterious consequences for her seriously ill child. As is the case for their mothers, children may realize for the first time the seriousness of their illness. The somatic distress associated with infections, fever, and mucous membrane irritations may precipitate that realization. Withdrawal by their mothers may further frighten the children, inducing feelings of loneliness or the feeling that they have been abandoned or written off. They may feel cut off from the one person with whom they could communicate their concerns about their future. Although some adults may fear that discussing death with children will heighten their anxiety, others suggest that conveying permission to discuss any aspect of illness can decrease children's feelings of isolation and loneliness (Waecheter 1971). We found that even when some mothers were in the child's immediate environment they tended not to talk to the child. Thus, withdrawal of mothers may precipitate or severely exacerbate emotional problems in their children.

THERAPEUTIC INTERVENTION

Our findings indicate that mothers are at risk for psychological problems when the child begins to show signs of drug toxicity. Alternatively, mothers could be considered to be at risk at all points of the treatment regimen. Therapeutic programs to assist mothers in coping with the stress of parenting a seriously ill child can take several forms: individual therapy, parent support groups, primary nurse or physician support relationships, and a variety of other mental health interventions. The relevance of psychiatric or psychosocial therapy programs for parents of ill children have not been scrupulously examined. However, findings from descriptive studies of how parents cope with serious childhood illness indicate possible approaches to designing programs for parents.

It is probable that the psychosocial adjustment of parents of children receiving treatment for cancer is related to the degree of support they feel they receive from their families, physicians, and other parents of ill children. These findings indicate that traditional mental health programs such as those offering psychotherapy may not be indicated for these parents. Rather, programs aimed at encouraging their spouses, families, and primary physicians to support parents through their crisis seems to be indicated. The best type of "support," however, is unclear. Support can range from simply encouraging a parent to communicate feelings to providing instrumental help with the ill child and with family activities. The most critical element is that relatives and caregivers are known to be available when parents feel they need emotional support.

Efforts to support parents during the course of a child's illness are a help not only during the illness but also during the parents' adaptation following the child's death. Spinetta, Swarner, and Sheposh (1981) found that those parents who were best adjusted after the death of a child appeared to have had support available prior to their child's death. Furthermore, parents who had provided the information and emotional support the child needed, and who had done so at a level consistent with the child's age and level of development, appeared better adjusted after the child's death.

In therapy programs designed to assist mothers to cope with the demands of parenting a seriously ill child, two goals seem essential. The first is to provide mothers with opportunities for developing supportive relationships with primary caregivers and other parents of ill children. Parent support groups such as the Candlelighters already exist in many communities. The primary caregivers should familiarize parents with the benefits of participating in these groups. The second goal is to encourage mothers to communicate openly with their children, possibly even about their own feelings. This, in turn, will give the children permission to communicate their own fears and concerns openly. This goal may be difficult to achieve, especially if the mother's personality style is inconsistent with discussing either her own feelings or those of her child. Learning to express feelings may be more effectively achieved in a one-to-one therapy situation. Both of these program goals are aimed at alleviating depression and anxiety in the mothers of seriously ill children. Prevention of these severe emotional crises may prevent mothers from withdrawing from their children at a time when the children are in need of so much nurturance, physical indulgence, and warmth.

REFERENCES

Binger, C. M., A. R., Albin, R. C. Feuerstein, J. H. Kushner, S. Zoger, and C. Mikkelsen. 1969. "Childhood Leukemia: Emotional Impact on Patient and Family." *New England Journal of Medicine* 280:414-418.
Goldfogel, L. 1972. "Working With the Parent of a Dying Child." In M. H. Browning and E. P. Lewis, eds. *The Dying Patient*. New York: The American Journal of Nursing Co.
Spinetta, J. J., J. A. Swarner, and J. P. Sheposh. 1981. "Effective Parental Coping Following the Death of a Child With Cancer." *Journal of Pediatric Psychology* 6:251-263.
Susman, E. J., A. R. Hollenbeck, E. D. Nannis, B. E. Strope, S. P. Hersh, A. S. Levine, and P. A. Pizzo. 1981. "The Impact of an Intensive Medical Regimen on the Social Behavior of Child and Adolescent Cancer Patients." *Journal of Applied Developmental Psychology* 2:29-47.
Waechter, E. A. 1971. "Children's Awareness of Fatal Illness." *American Journal of Nursing* 71:1168-1172.

Suffering by Children:
Some Observations of Brave
Children and Their Families
at a Children's Hospital

Steven N. Sparta

Cassell (1982) has made an important distinction between suffering and physical distress, asserting that suffering is experienced by persons, not merely bodies, and is related to the challenges to the person as a social or psychological entity. According to this view, it is the responsibility of the treating professional to recognize and deal with the fact that there is much more to illness than physical pain.

I have seen this lesson illustrated when children present surface symptoms of abdominal pain, respiratory difficulties, or secondary complications caused by their failure to take sufficient care of themselves. These problems, which have brought the patients to medical care, may actually represent grief, anxiety, loneliness, or the frustration of unfulfilled dreams stemming from their lack of resolution of the consequences of past illnesses. When such complaints are heard in the absence of verifiable organic etiology and in the resulting absence of prescribed medical treatment, these patients may be considered troublesome or difficult. Sometimes health professionals avoid the true meaning of these patients' complaints, angrily believing that their valuable time is being diverted from care of the "truly" sick. Ignoring the dimension of suffering, however, can

Steven N. Sparta, PhD, is Chief Psychologist at the Children's Hospital, San Diego, and is Associate Clinical Professor of Psychiatry, University of California at San Diego, San Diego, CA.

© 1988 by The Haworth Press, Inc. All rights reserved.

produce stress that creates organic vulnerability and eventually gives way to the presence of disease.

Children can and do suffer, although their suffering is often masked or is communicated in nonadult terms that go unrecognized. All of the caveats about recognition and treatment of adult suffering are compounded by children's various developmental "languages," which health care professionals may not know. This article examines situations involving childhood cancer, progressive muscular dystrophy, sexual abuse, and prolonged hospitalization, with particular emphasis on the presence of suffering in children and the ways in which it is communicated.

One aspect of suffering relates to the dimension of expectancy, which is crucial in establishing a child's sense of underlying psychological stability, and thus in preventing or reducing suffering. A disease often presents a course of an unstable, and thus confusing, set of expectations for the future. "What is happening to me inside my body, where I can't see?"; "I don't see anything wrong, but I had to miss school and go to appointments with the doctor"; "It seems each time I have one kind of thing explained, after it's finished another thing happens — maybe I can never be sure of what might happen next." The role of expectancy is known to be a key variable in predicting children's feelings and motivations. What the professional or parent explains to a child usually has implications for the expectancy that is developed. For this particular reason, hospitals prepare children for surgery or hospitalization by offering concrete information in a safe environment, ordered in appropriate sequential fashion, and using language that is appropriate to the individual child's age.

Especially with children, much communication is nonverbal, reflecting the expression, "It's not what you say but how you say it that counts." Thus, what adults conclude, in terms of their religious, psychological, social, and medical understanding, about a child's illness has profound implications for their communication with the child about the illness. Openness and attention to the level of the child's understanding (including the child's concepts of death), as well as the adults' own coming-to-terms with values of life and death, must all be faced in communicating with the child. Parents who are not attuned to these issues must recognize the likelihood that the child will develop attitudes and expectations that are derived from what they discern of how the parents *feel*, regardless of what they choose to *say*.

When children are hospitalized, particularly for long times, their suffering can easily be overlooked because of the dramatic nature of injections, painful or distasteful treatments, bleeding, pain, use of advanced technological instruments, and so on, which demand acute attention. Sometimes parents must be strong for the child because the future is all too painfully predictable and known. Once, when visiting a school in the San Diego area, I was told of two brothers who had Duchennes muscular dystrophy. The younger boy, aware of the progressive and ultimately lethal course of the disease, saw his own future physical functioning in his older brother's. In addition to the loss of physical ability, there would undoubtedly be continual change in his identity as he became progressively weaker and more helpless. The younger boy's suffering can be better explained in terms of his expectations of helplessness and loss than in the measurement of his existing degree of physical limitation.

For young children, separation from family represents a loss of self as frightening and devastating as any of the physical procedures they endure. In the developmental process of individuation and separation, the child attempts to evolve an intrapsychic self made up of perceptions, reasoning, and memories that are different from those of all other persons. The ego functions grow from the development of individuation. In the process of separation, the child, through guided positive experience, is helped to achieve distance from the primary caretaking figure, to formulate boundaries, and to disengage from the mother in a process that established relations with other people. These "people-objects" become symbolic representations that the child uses throughout life.

Differentiation begins between the ages of four to eight months; a practice period occurs from eight to twenty months; a rapprochement phase lasts for up to two years, and so on. During the transitions from one period to another, the child faces a particular challenge through which he or she can experience relative psychic discomfort and pain. The process of illness or hospitalization represents a fundamental threat to this developmental course. Children faced with the stressors of illness find it much more difficult to see themselves as independent from the family. The health care professional can view suffering as a consequence of the threat of disruption to this natural developmental progression toward mastery. When parents have to leave the hospital or cannot be present all of the time the child is in the hospital, the child's suffering changes because his or her internal stability as an individual is threatened.

Children must also contend with physical illness with an immature set of cognitive abilities. Difficult physical, philosophical, religious, and psychological challenges (such as understanding the concept of death) can be bewildering to children, who have fewer intellectual tools and who are more dependent on others than adults. This is not to suggest that children are unaware of death; indeed, increasing evidence shows that children as young as five and six years understand death along multiple lines of comprehension. However, attention must still be paid to appropriate attempts at communicating with children in a manner that does not overwhelm them with complexity or avoid the content that children can hear and deserve to hear.

In my experience with children being treated for serious illnesses such as cancer or muscular dystrophy, it is the pending destruction of personhood that presents the major threat to well-being. The more obviously painful side effects of radiation, medication, injections, and so on play a role that receives some recognition and for which there is potential assistance, and do so almost to the exclusion of the negative self-ascriptions the child makes in everyday family or social life. The physical side effects are observed first and dominate simply because they are so visible and because, indeed, they vicariously wound the observer as well. However, the child's helplessness, the uncertainty of disease and treatment outcome, and the impact on the balance of the family system are all in intricate interplay in the development and maintenance of suffering beyond the physical side effects. In addition, the vicarious suffering that parents experience can make the debilitating side effects more severe and can possibly create a feedback loop between the child and the family. Thus, the understanding of suffering in children must, by definition, take into account the influence of their siblings and parents on their emotions.

A respirator-dependent adolescent girl with severe muscle weakness was recurrently hospitalized for infection. She could barely speak — and, when she did, her voice was scarcely above a whisper — and she appeared to be severely undernourished. Considering the rush to stabilize her medical condition and the constant care she required, it was ironic that a person given so much attention was so psychologically alone. The patient was finally referred to me when it was discovered that she could not sleep. Sleep deprivation resulted in total exhaustion. During the initial psychological consultation about her sleep disturbance, it became obvious that she was a poignant illustration of the silent, powerful effects of suffering, which had a clearly observable bearing on her medical course. From further bedside consultation there emerged the picture of a severely emotionally isolated, depressed youngster who was afraid that she would die if she relinquished conscious control of her breathing at night. In addition, her family was equally debilitated by their own pain and a coping pattern of avoidance. Because of the patient's great difficulty in speaking, written exchanges were necessary. Her letters (Figure 1) were simple and to the point, and they attested to a great quantity of unexpressed feelings. It bears remembering that although her fears were intense, they had gone unrecognized for many months or longer, and information about them was not elicited without inquiry. Fear of death and feelings of social isolation, interpersonal distance, frustration, and guilt were all conveyed in the patient's brief but poignant messages.

When children have been sexually abused, hospital staff are, of course, rightfully horrified. Much attention is focused on the sexual act itself, but how can the cause of suffering be observed? In addition to the physical pain that may have occurred at the time of the act, there are other dimensions relating to "physical distress outside the realm of bodies." For sexually abused children, these dimensions frequently include fear of reprisal after they have divulged the abuse; embarrassment or self-condemnation about having been a party to the "terribly bad" thing that is referred to so often by sympathetic adults; and concern that their bodies are different, damaged, or irrevocably altered in some mysterious way.

Although adults tend to interpret the events primarily from the developmental perspective of sexuality and its consequences for

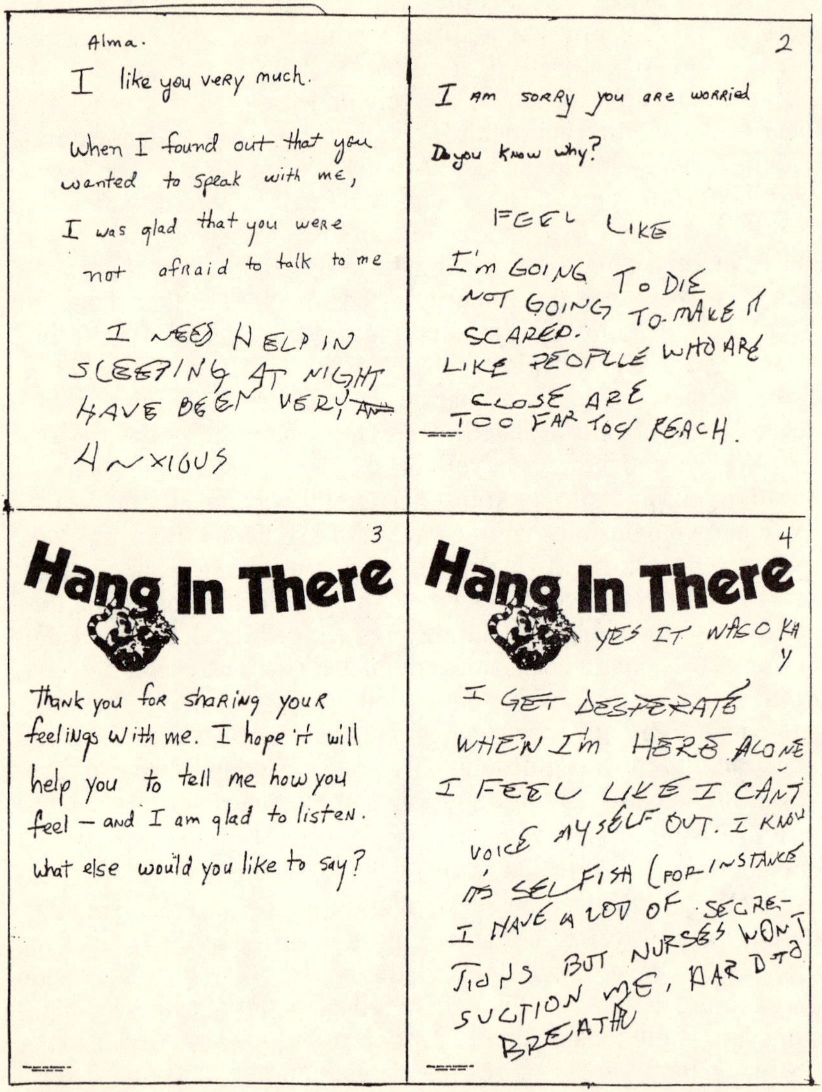

Alma.

I like you very much.

When I found out that you wanted to speak with me,

I was glad that you were not afraid to talk to me

I NEED HELP IN SLEEPING AT NIGHT HAVE BEEN VERY ANXIOUS

2

I AM SORRY you are worried

Do you know why?

FEEL LIKE

I'm GOING TO DIE NOT GOING TO MAKE IT SCARED. LIKE PEOPLE WHO ARE CLOSE ARE TOO FAR TO REACH.

3

Hang In There

Thank you for sharing your feelings with me. I hope it will help you to tell me how you feel — and I am glad to listen. What else would you like to say?

4

Hang In There

YES IT WAS OKAY

I GET DESPERATE WHEN I'm HERE ALONE I FEEL LIKE I CAN'T VOICE MYSELF OUT. I KNOW IT'S SELFISH (FOR INSTANCE I HAVE A LOT OF SECRETIONS BUT NURSES WON'T SUCTION ME, HARD TO BREATH

FIGURE 1. Copies of patient's letters written as part of psychological therapy.

identity, another particularly devastating aspect of these cases is the violation of trust between a dependent child and an adult authority figure, who frequently is not only known to the child but is even a family member. In such situations, adults frequently do not recognize the children's emotions and the children self-protectively will not volunteer them.

One five-and-a-half-year-old boy who, within one year, had been repeatedly molested by his adoptive stepfather, would not confirm to the police or his mother the details of what had occurred. Only through physical examination was there any possibility of corroborating the story of abuse. Suffering in cases like this one takes the form of anger against exploitation and vulnerability, as shown in Figure 2. In this drawing, the boy engaged in significant discharge of affect in relating the intense anger he felt toward his adoptive father, portraying it by what seems to be vague scribbling that includes an ax with which he wanted to attack this man.

In other cases of abuse, suffering may be understood to come not from physical injury to the child's body but from the manipulation of fear by perpetrators who threaten to harm the child or the child's family if the child divulges the "secret." In still other cases, suffering arises from the manipulation of psychological need. For example, the molester of a four-and-a-half-year-old fatherless boy told the boy that *he* was his father — a statement that the child readily and fully believed. In no case can the physical act of sexual abuse be ignored, but many more questions must be recognized and exposed if the meaning of the child's suffering is to be dealt with sufficiently in an adaptational fashion.

Another dimension of children's suffering has to do with the concept of role. Everyone has a role in life, and children have their roles, as sons, daughters, siblings, or students. In some respects, not having highly developed roles is easier for children, as they may experience less psychological dissonance when they are out of role. Nonetheless, illness changes a child's role. For example, school attendance is frequently reduced or eliminated entirely, isolating the child from peers and the classroom and resulting in major losses in a source of the child's social functioning. The child is diminished by that loss. In conscious recognition of the importance of the child's

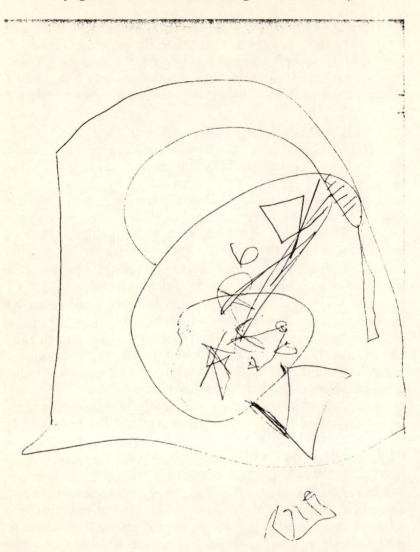

FIGURE 2. Drawing done by a boy who had been sexually abused by his adoptive father. In this picture, the boy revealed intense anger: within what appears to be vague scribbling is an ax with which he wanted to attack his adoptive father.

concept of role, all children's hospitals should, as many already do, attempt to have on-site schoolrooms.

Suffering seems to be affected by the extent to which there is a network of belonging. Everyone can and does belong to larger groups. For children, the primary larger group is the family, but there are others, including school sports teams, neighborhood groups, the extended family, and so on. Without these relations to others, a child's emotions will not find expression. Children who suffer from prolonged illnesses or who have been seriously uprooted by changes in their lives suffer from isolation from their previous group activities. The role of the family becomes more important to such children, but bewildered parents may be unable to act in an entirely familiar, consistent fashion.

Awareness of the dimension of suffering in ill children also demands attention to children's concepts of their bodies. Before people develop the higher-order intellectual abilities that enable them to reflect on themselves and to think about the world in abstract terms, they must first have a sense of self as a body state. In childhood, the ego does not differentiate between self and others, creating a world that becomes a simultaneously thinking-and-feeling state. When a child's body is disfigured, examined, or changed in any way, this may be a terribly frightening obstacle to the developmental struggle to understand and cope with all other areas.

Communication with the suffering child is the basis for both diagnosis and treatment. Suffering is frequently inferred from children's overt acts, but real understanding of this dimension is more subtle and complex. Children's withdrawal, sadness, anger, loneliness, and frustration can be mistakenly attributed to, for example, "the needles," rather than their changed relationships with others and with their own bodies, their sense of instability, or their inability to predict the future reliably. For this reason, communication with children about their suffering should employ many modes of expression that are responsive to the child, such as the use of play or drawings. We know that children are intrinsically motivated to draw, that their drawings depict their perceptions of themselves, and that drawings are a medium for communicating internal feeling states that they have difficulty putting into words.

Figure 3, by a ten-year-old leukemia patient, depicts a markedly

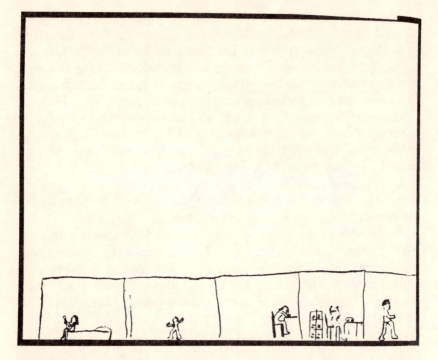

FIGURE 3. This drawing was done by a ten-year-old male leukemia patient on chemotherapy, in remission, 27 months from diagnosis. Among the items scored as maladaptive in this drawing are the amount of paper used, total compartmentalization, the presence of barriers between all the family members, the absence of color, the absence of faces, and the body positions of the figures. This drawing received a score of 19.

From Spinetta, J. J., H. H. McLaren, R. W. Fox, and S. Sparta, "Kinetic Family Drawing in Childhood Cancer: A Revised Application of an Age-Dependent Measure." In J. J. Spinetta and P. Deasy Spinetta, eds. *Living with Childhood Cancer*, St. Louis: C. V. Mosby, p. 109.

different emotional tone than the drawing shown in Figure 4, by the mother of a ten-year-old leukemia patient. From a sophisticated scoring system of kinetic family drawing developed by Spinetta et al. (1981), communication, self-image, and emotional tone can be scored along nineteen separate dimensions. The natural course of expression of suffering is such that content of this kind is frequently

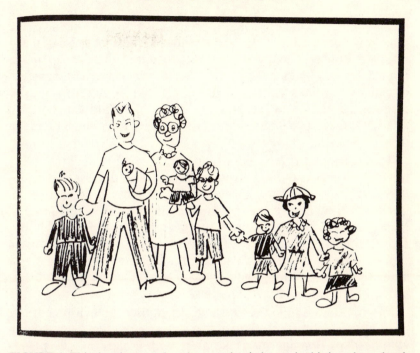

FIGURE 4. This drawing was done by a mother in her early thirties whose daughter is a ten-year-old leukemia patient, in relapse, on chemotherapy, 81 months from diagnosis. The judge rates this drawing as adaptive in such items as lack of compartmentalization and barriers. The figures are standing, facing forward, and mostly complete. Also note that many colors were used and a large amount of space was used. The total score given is 4.

From Spinetta, J. J., H. H. McLaren, R. W. Fox, and S. Sparta, "Kinetic Family Drawing in Childhood Cancer: A Revised Application of an Age-Dependent Measure." In J. J. Spinetta and P. Deasy Spinetta, eds. *Living with Childhood Cancer*, St. Louis: C. V. Mosby, p. 116.

encountered in drawings when conversation has been of limited value.

Although I have reviewed ways to recognize children's suffering, there are important reasons why it is difficult to do so. One reason is that awareness of children's suffering is painful indeed. It is quite understandable that caretakers who are struggling to contend with their own grief over a child's condition may show repression or denial. It is seductively easy to prefer quieter, more passive and withdrawn children to those who scream and plead because of physical pain, although it may be the quieter children who are experiencing deeper loneliness and despair. Precisely because of this aspect of caregiving, the suffering of quieter children is more likely to be forgotten. Adults who recognize suffering in a child experience it intensely; they have internalized responsibility for a much more dependent human.

Through initial investment of time in listening to children, additional problems can be prevented and levels of distress can be reduced. The caregiver can always choose, in a psychological sense, how to deal with even the most tragic circumstances. All psychotherapy strives for the attainment of greater personal responsibility, recognizing its relevance by describing feeling states that can be characterized as "suffering" states. It is these inner states that best allow the identification, understanding, and alleviation of the suffering of children and their families.

In what Cassel (1982) has called the transcendental dimension, bonding with something larger than oneself is crucial for coping with despair. Bonding may take place with groups or concepts related to the human community's ideals or to God. In researching the subject of suffering, many of my sources led to literature in the fields of religion and philosophy. The word *suffering* is sometimes difficult to find in the psychological and psychiatric literature, no doubt because of the difficulties in applying empirical techniques or the scientific method to the concept. I am reminded of my conversation in 1980 with the psychologist Dr. Bruno Bettelheim, who related how crucial transcendental belief had been in differentiating between those who had survived the concentration camp experience and those who had not.

Another point about children's suffering is that children not only endure suffering but sometimes do so in a way that is inspiring and that advances their personal development. We find that the developmental challenges that are posed when children are hospitalized can be overcome, and these children can derive a new sense of security or trust in their inner resources. Such attitudes not only are beneficial in their coping with illness, but extend to almost all other areas of their lives. Spinetta et al. (1981:4) have written about the experi-

ences of children with cancer in a manner that expresses the courage
I have often observed among suffering children and their families:

> The child offers an example of the determination to live fully
> and well even against overwhelming odds. Even the child who
> must die at a young age can further the human potential. Those
> children who live, and their numbers are growing, are teach-
> ing us that a little body can contain a powerful fighter, a strug-
> gler, an individual who is determined to show that life is worth
> living to the fullest and that one must continue to fight for life
> even in the face of great handicaps, and from the children who
> have died, we have learned that the most powerful weapon
> against certain death is the will to live life fully in the face of
> that death.

REFERENCES

Cassel, E. J. 1982. "The Nature of Suffering and the Goals of Medicine." *New England Journal of Medicine* 306(11):639-645.
Spinetta, J., H. H. McLaren, R. W. Fox, and S. Sparta. 1981. "The Kinetic Family Drawing in Childhood Cancer: A Revised Application of an Age-Inde- pendent Measure." In J. J. Spinetta and P. Spinetta, eds. *Living with Child- hood Cancer*. St. Louis, MO: C. V. Mosby, pp. 86-121.

The Needs of Sarcoma Patients from Diagnosis Through Follow-Up

Joan Kaiser

Treatment for a malignant tumor is complicated and difficult. It usually includes preoperative chemotherapy and surgical ablation of the neoplasm, either by limb salvage or, if this is not possible, by amputation. After surgery the patient will usually continue to receive adjuvant chemotherapy for six months or longer. Patients who have radiosensitive tumors will also receive radiation therapy as part of their treatment protocol.

Patients must be carefully evaluated before limb salvage surgery can be contemplated. This is a highly stressful time for them. Patients are often referred from other hospitals for limb-sparing treatment, and their expectations run high, balanced by anxiety about failing to meet the criteria, which include the following: (1) that the patient has reached skeletal maturity or has nearly done so; (2) that there is not extensive tumor involvement in soft tissue; (3) that an arteriogram does not reveal arterial invasion or compromise; and (4) that if preoperative chemotherapy is to be administered to decrease the tumor mass, the patient can physically tolerate this treatment. (In some institutions, preoperative chemotherapy is not administered.)

During the work-up period, patients often comment on the supportiveness of members of the health care team. This may be in contrast to their previous experience in a community hospital setting, where they may have been viewed with pity because of their age and diagnosis and where many people, including physicians and nurses, spent minimal time with them.

Joan Kaiser, RN, MA, Staff Development, Good Samaritan Hospital, Suffern, NY.

© 1988 by The Haworth Press, Inc. All rights reserved.

Before surgery is performed, be it amputation or a limb preserv-
ing procedure, preoperative chemotherapy may be given. This is
done to shrink the primary tumor, destroy pulmonary metastases,
and, in cases of osteogenic sarcoma, to evaluate tumor destruction
by histological review of the specimen at the time of definitive surgery. Patients and families often worry that the tumor will not respond to chemotherapy, which might rule out limb salvage. For
many patients and families, it is much easier to focus on saving the
limb than on the diagnosis of cancer, with its terrifying implications.

Patients also fear that if they do not respond to one chemotherapy
protocol, they may not respond to another, and that nothing further
will then be available. This is sometimes the case. Patients who
receive chemotherapy for primary bone tumors have the opportunity to meet peers in the physician's office or the hospital clinic,
and they have all seen patients for whom one chemotherapy protocol has failed and who have then been switched to another protocol.
Even more worrisome, they have seen patients who have been
"cured" of cancer, only to have a local recurrence or metastases at
a later time and for whom all chemotherapy has then failed. Failure
is more likely in this situation because recurrent lesions are usually
more resistant to chemotherapy than the original tumor was.

Once a patient has been diagnosed as having a primary bone tumor and has had an open biopsy, the bone containing the neoplasm
is at increased risk for fracture because its structure has been weak-
ened. These patients are instructed to walk with crutches to avoid
weight bearing, and may be fitted with a long leg brace for further
protection. They are told that a fracture would diminish the possibility of cure because it increases hematogenous dissemination of
the tumor, and could mean that amputation will be required. If a
fracture occurs, surrounding tissue will be contaminated by tumor
cells, which are spread by the hematoma that forms at the fracture
site. Many adolescents cope with the fear of fracture and amputation by risk-taking behavior — they sometimes refuse to use crutches,
will not wear a brace, and, in effect, totally deny that a potential
problem exists.

Patients who are to undergo chemotherapy understand that they
will be receiving highly toxic drugs to manage a life-threatening

tumor. A great amount of responsibility is placed on them, and they and their families require intensive education in order to participate freely in this aspect of the treatment plan. All of the side effects related to the chemotherapeutic drugs that the patient will receive are spelled out. Even a brief list of these side effects provides a sense of the overpowering amount of information that patients receive. This list, which is part of the informed consent form that patients are usually required to sign, includes alopecia; nausea and vomiting; stomatitis; pancytopenia; nephrotoxicity; skin hypersensitivity, especially after sun exposure; neurological changes; peripheral neuropathies, such as pain, numbness, tingling, and loss of motion in an extremity; jaw and joint pain; paralytic ilius; hemorrhagic cystitis, a result of irritation of the lining of the bladder by chemotherapy by-products; cardiac toxicity; pulmonary fibrosis; sterility; ototoxicity; and spontaneous pneumothorax from necrotic pulmonary nodules. Despite the fact that the patient knows that these toxicities will not happen all at once and that not all of them may occur, it is an overwhelming list.

Patients become closely involved in their treatment program. They calculate their intake and output and are aware, for example, that cyclophosphamide (Cytoxan) can cause hemorrhagic cystitis, so that they must force fluids and wake up once during the night to void in order to prevent waste products from remaining in the bladder, or that cis-platinum (Platinol) can cause renal failure, so that they must be well hydrated before and during treatment. In some instances, platinum is given on an outpatient basis or in a day hospital setting. This means that patients are required to hydrate themselves orally before coming in for chemotherapy.

Patients who are receiving high-dose Methotrexate are taught that this cytotoxic agent will cause them fewer renal problems than some other agents and is best excreted in an alkaline urine. They are given sodium bicarbonate tablets, are taught to check their urine pH after voiding, and to take additional bicarbonate if the pH drops to 7 or less.

With the knowledge that chemotherapy may cause pancytopenia, patients are particularly aware of their blood counts. They are instructed to avoid crowds and ill people if their white blood count falls below 2,000. They may need to be hospitalized if the white blood count continues to drop and they become septic, which is always a possibility. Immunosuppressed patients are also cautioned to avoid children with chicken pox, which could be lethal for them. Patients are also instructed in proper precautions to take if their platelet count drops below 40,000.

These are a few examples of the kinds of information that patients receive before and during chemotherapy. After several courses of chemotherapy, it is time for surgical ablation of the tumor. For patients who are to undergo amputation, a rigorous rehabilitation program is begun preoperatively and is resumed three to four days after the amputation.

Patients who undergo limb salvage surgery spend longer periods in bed — as much as three or four weeks. During the first few days, patients may be preoccupied with whether the tumor margins (surgical margins) are free of tumor (negative) or contaminated (positive), but generally they are greatly relieved to have completed the surgical portion of their treatment. Some patients will require further surgery, in the form of thoracotomy and wedge resection to resect pulmonary nodules, but they tend not to focus on the chance that an amputation may still be necessary.

Patients often have a great deal of pain after limb salvage surgery. Their mobility is also limited, especially if lower extremity surgery has been done. A proximal femur resection requires the patient to lie relatively flat with the head of the bed elevated to not more than thirty degrees. This provides the support that the resected muscle groups previously provided and is necessary in order to avoid dislocation of the hip joint until scar tissue has formed. Bed rest may continue for two weeks or more. Early mobility may be achieved with an abduction brace containing a thigh cuff and pelvic band, which supports the leg as the patient turns to the other side. During bed rest, the patient is vulnerable to all of the complications of immobility and must be monitored for respiratory compromise, pulmonary emboli, anorexia, constipation, formation of renal calculi, decubiti, and loss of muscle tone. A bed rehabilitation program, respiratory exercises, and a balanced diet with plenty of fluids are all important.

It is equally important for caregivers to plan time with these patients, encouraging them to talk about how they are dealing with this phase of the treatment course. Patients may be fearful of the rehabilitation program and wonder how, if they feel so weak right now, they will ever become ambulatory. In dealing with patients' anxieties at this time, it is immensely helpful to provide them with encouragement, to clarify the purpose of a bed physical therapy program, and to remind them of other patients who have undergone the same or similar surgery and are now fully mobile.

Once the surgical wound is sufficiently healed, chemotherapy is reinstated. It is important to wait for evidence that the wound is healing successfully because premature resumption of chemotherapy or radiation therapy can cause the wound to fall apart and become infected. Because infected tissue around metal cannot heal, the implant might then have to be removed and the patient treated for six weeks with intravenous antibiotics before a new implant can be inserted. If an allograft has been inserted, it is especially important to wait for evidence of good wound healing, since the rate of infection in the presence of preoperative chemotherapy and allograft insertion tends to be higher than among patients with metal implants.

Once chemotherapy is resumed after surgery, it continues for three to six months. After chemotherapy has been completed, frequent follow-up is necessary, first every two to three months and then every six months, to ensure that the patient has remained disease-free or to detect metastases or local recurrences at an early stage. The follow-up visits remind patients that they are still considered cancer patients, even if they see themselves as cured. Long-term follow-up is important, although if a recurrence does not appear within two to three years it is not likely to do so.

Throughout treatment, patients can be expected to have various needs. As Fedora (1985), an oncology nurse who underwent successful treatment for osteogenic sarcoma, defined these needs, they include the need for information, for honest expression, for acceptance and understanding, for peer support, and for normalcy.

Need for Information. Fear of the unknown gives rise to increased anxiety. Most patients want detailed information about procedures, test results, treatment plans, and expected outcomes. Supplying this information increases patients' security and sense of control, as does including them in decision making. By taking cues from patients, staff can supply them with the type and amount of information they are seeking without overwhelming them.

Need for Honest Expression. Patients' emotions are varied, and include anger, fear, resentment, disbelief, guilt, depression, and confusion. Patients need someone they can trust to whom they can express these emotions honestly and without being judged. Empathetic nurses can provide time for patients to verbalize their feelings and to receive accurate information along with psychological support. This helps them through emotional turmoil, helps them reestablish priorities among their values, and helps them regain a sense of mental equilibrium.

Need for Acceptance and Understanding. Patients need an atmosphere that is characterized by these qualities in order to express their feelings freely without fear of being rejected or becoming isolated from the health care team. Patients closely watch the health care team, friends, and family for signs of repugnance when they see their alopecia or amputated stump. Family acceptance increases patients' self-esteem, self-acceptance, and self-confidence. Patients also need to feel acceptance and understanding when they "lose it" during stressful situations—for example, when a new site cannot be found for insertion of an intravenous line, when they are waiting for test reports that will indicate whether or not they are free of disease, or when they learn that they have developed metastases.

Need for Peer Support. As patients share their failures and triumphs, whether in a group setting or informally, they lend and receive support and provide ideas for others who are undergoing similar surgery and treatments. As patients begin to see that they are not alone and that others are struggling to deal with issues that are similar to the ones they confront, sharing groups can be invaluable. Groups can include present inpatients and volunteer patients who are still receiving treatment on an outpatient basis or who have completed therapy and have resumed their normal lives and activities.

Need for Normalcy. Becoming a patient sometimes means that one's previous identity has been lost and creates the need to find oneself again. This may involve reawakening some personality characteristics and regaining a sense of independence. Patients begin to realize the need to mobilize positive forces as a necessary step toward full recovery. Staff can help patients regain a sense of normalcy by providing means for them to socialize within the hospital environment, where common issues such as families, backgrounds, and interests can be discussed.

In conclusion, treatment for a malignant bone or soft-tissue sarcoma is complicated and difficult. Because the disciplines of surgery, chemotherapy, and radiation therapy may all be involved, each affecting the special needs of these patients, nursing management of this patient population requires many skills.

REFERENCE

Fedora, N. 1985. "Fighting for My Leg . . . and My Life." *Orthopaedic Nursing* 4:39-42.

BIBLIOGRAPHY

Aiken, S. 1982. "Family Structure and Utilization of Cancer Support Groups." *Oncology Nursing Forum* 9:22-26.

Boren, H. 1985. "Adolescent Adjustment to Amputation Necessitated by Bone Cancer." *Orthopaedic Nursing* 4:30-32.

Fountain, M. 1985. "Psychosocial Support for the Person Experiencing Cancer." *Orthopaedic Nursing* 4:33-35.

Kagen, L. 1976. "Use of Denial in Adolescents with Bone Cancer." *Health and Social Work* 1:71-86.

Kagen-Goodheart, L. 1977. "Reentry: Living with Childhood Cancer." *American Journal of Orthopsychiatry* 47:651-658.

Lansky, S. 1985. "Impediments to Treatment and Rehabilitation of the Childhood Cancer Patient." *Ca – A Cancer Journal for Clinicians* 35:302-307.

Nirenberg, A. 1985. "The Adolescent with Osteogenic Sarcoma." *Orthopaedic Nursing* 4:11-15.

Tebbi, C. et al. 1985. "The Role of Social Support Systems in Adolescent Cancer Amputees." *Cancer* 56:965-971.

Walters, J. 1981. "Coping with a Leg Amputation." *American Journal of Nursing* 81:1349-1352.

Wilbur, J. 1980. "Sexual Development and Body Image in the Teenager with Cancer." *Frontiers in Radiation Therapy and Oncology* 14:108-114.

Treatment of Fractures
in Children with Malignancies

David Price Roye, Jr.

Children who are undergoing treatment for malignant tumors are at a fairly high risk for pathological fractures. An important example is the child with leukemia who is undergoing chemotherapy. These children are frequently given high-dose steroids, which may lead to rather severe osteopenia. The fact that the children are ill, not weight-bearing, and, in some circumstances, not getting proper nutrition may contribute to the osteopenia. This particular set of circumstances can lead to easy fracture of long bones, particularly in the lower extremities. The child may step off on the leg and have pain in the ankle, and subsequent radiographs may reveal a buckle fracture of the distal tibia. An example is the patient who, after being released after prolonged hospitalization for relapse of leukemia, falls on the same day and sustains a displaced femur fracture.

In addition to pathologic fractures caused by osteoporosis, fractures may occur through destructive lesions in bone caused by the malignancy itself. Fractures through destructive lesions may cause pain, swelling, and difficulty with ambulation even when they are nondisplaced. It is important to know that these fractures are common and are sustained partially as a result of the treatment. If there is swelling or pain in an extremity, fracture should be suspected even when the patient reports no important trauma. In addition, it is important from an orthopedic point of view not to overtreat these children. Fractures that have occurred in osteopenic bone will heal at a normal rate despite osteoporosis. Therefore, they do not need any more vigorous treatment than a similarly displaced fracture in a

David Price Roye, Jr., MD, is Assistant Professor of Orthopedic Surgery, College of Physicians and Surgeons, Columbia University, New York, NY.

© 1988 by The Haworth Press, Inc. All rights reserved.

child who does not have systemic disease. In fact, since the child is already limited by the disease and perhaps by a general malaise, overtreatment can further diminish the child's ability to walk and stand and maintain motion; in fact, overtreatment may create more problems than the fracture alone would have.

Because every situation is different, it is not possible to formulate specific guidelines but, in general, we recommend first that casting for complete fractures be lightweight and form-fitting in order to allow as much function as possible. When at all possible, weight-bearing on the cast should be encouraged to encourage incorporation of mineralized bone, and casts should be removed early. Again, when possible, simple posterior splints should be used to allow regular ranging of the adjacent joints. In a situation in which possible instability precludes complete removal of a cast—for example, midshaft tibia fracture—a functional brace can be manufactured to allow the child to return to more normal activity faster.

Another consideration in these fractures is the possible surgical treatment of displaced long-bone fractures. In children who have a reasonably good prognosis and who have sustained a femur fracture through nonpathologic bone—that is, bone in which there is no tumor involvement—surgery may be indicated. Although cast treatment is the most common form of treatment for children's long bone fractures, surgery offers a way of providing immediate stability and allowing the children to return immediately to nearly full function. Surgery can prevent the need for the child to endure prolonged bed rest and prolonged casting and can allow more functional recovery. Again, the indication for these surgical interventions is individual.

When fractures occur through pathological bone, it is frequently necessary to treat the tumor itself. This, of course, depends entirely on the histological type of tumor: some tumors respond to chemotherapy, some to radiation, some to combinations of these two treatments. During the medical treatment of the malignancy at the site of the fracture, treatment of the fracture should be instituted using the principles outlined.

Advantage of Early Spinal Stabilization and Fusion in Patients with Duchenne Muscular Dystrophy

Michael D. Sussman

During their preteen and early teenage years, 50 to 80 percent of patients with Duchenne muscular dystrophy will develop a severe collapsing type of scoliosis (Gibson et al. 1978; Renshaw 1982; Robin 1977), usually with the convexity toward the side of the dominant hand (Johnson and Yarness 1976). This spinal deformity will cause decreased sitting tolerance and comfort, thereby diminishing the quality of these patients' lives. With each ten-degree increase in scoliosis, vital capacity is diminished by 4 percent in addition to the 4 percent loss per year owing to the progressive muscle weakness associated with their muscular dystrophy (Kurz et al. 1983).

Various techniques have been advocated to prevent or retard the progression of spinal deformity in these patients. Seigel (1977) has recommended release of the rectus femoris and fascia lata, which he feels will decrease the asymmetry about the pelvis and thus reduce the chance of severe scoliosis. Milwaukee bracing has been tried and abandoned because muscular dystrophy patients do not tolerate these braces well (Robin 1977). A variety of underarm orthoses (TLSO) have been used; however, a recent review of the efficacy of orthoses has demonstrated that they are only capable of slowing the progression of curvatures below twenty-five degrees, and have little or no effect on curvatures above this magnitude (Hsu et al. 1982).

Michael D. Sussman, MD, is affiliated with the Department of Pediatrics, Children's Rehabilitation Center, University of Virginia School of Medicine, Charlottesville, VA.

© 1988 by The Haworth Press, Inc. All rights reserved.

105

Because of their dissatisfaction with bracing, Gibson et al. (1978) developed a custom seating system that is able to retard the progression of curvatures but, like orthoses, cannot prevent this progression from occurring.

Harrington instrumentation with spinal fusion has been advocated for patients whose curvatures are progressive and uncontrollable by external support (Bunch 1974; Gibson et al. 1978; Robin 1977; Sakai et al. 1977; Swank, Brown, and Perry 1982; Taddonio 1982). Although patients undergoing this procedure have done well on long-term follow-up, Harrington instrumentation, particularly in patients with osteopenic bone, requires supplemental external support until the fusion is solid and flattening of the spine in the sagittal plane is produced by Harrington distraction rods. The segmental spinal instrumentation technique of Luque has, in recent years, replaced the Harrington system for stabilization of neuromuscular spinal deformities (Herring and Wenger 1982; Sullivan and Conner 1982; Taddonio 1982). I have reviewed my experience during the past seven years with surgical treatment of the spinal deformity in eleven patients with Duchenne muscular dystrophy, with emphasis on these patients' perioperative course.

METHODS

I operated on all of the patients in this series, managed their postoperative care, and followed them at the Muscular Dystrophy Clinic at the Children's Rehabilitation Center of the University of Virginia. Patients were studied retrospectively and fell into three groups.

Group I: Between 1975 and 1980, the three patients in this group underwent posterior spine fusion with Harrington instrumentation from the upper thoracic spine to the sacrum. The mean age of these patients was thirteen years and nine months; their preoperative curvatures averaged sixty-nine degrees and their vital capacity was 54 percent of predicted. Preoperative radiographs in this group were not adequate to measure pelvic obliquity.

Group II: This group consists of the first three patients who underwent spinal fusion with Luque instrumentation in our clinic in 1980-81. The mean age of this group was fourteen years and eleven months. All of these patients had preoperative curvatures greater than seventy degrees; their mean preoperative curvature was eighty-two degrees and the mean. The mean preoperative pelvic obliquity among these patients, as measured by the angle of the intercrest line with a horizontal, was twenty-seven degrees. The mean preoperative vital capacity was 38 percent of predicted.

Group III: The five patients in this group underwent segmental spinal instrumentation with fusion after 1982. These patients had had surgery earlier in the course of their disease, when their curvatures were milder and their pulmonary function had deteriorated to a lesser degree than that of the patients in Group II. The average age of these patients was thirteen years and three months, with a range from ten years and four months to sixteen years. The mean preoperative curvature was forty-six degrees and pelvic obliquity was ten degrees. The mean preoperative vital capacity was 66 percent of predicted.

Surgical Techniques

For Group I patients, standard techniques for Harrington instrumentation were used, with fixation extending from the upper thoracic spine to the sacral ala using a sacral alar hook. In order to achieve fusion, facetectomy and decortication were done. Autogenous pelvic bone supplemented with bone from banked femoral heads was used as graft material. Postoperatively, patients were maintained on a regular hospital bed and allowed to log-roll only until they were fitted with a cast or orthoplast TLSO at the end of the first postoperative week, at which time sitting was allowed.

For patients in Groups II and III, the technique of segmental spinal instrumentation used was similar to that described by Luque (1982) and others (Allen and Ferguson 1982; Luque and Cardoso 1976). Two "L" rods were used, which were contoured to accommodate the residual scoliosis after manual intraoperative correction, as well as to impart lumbar lordosis and thoracic kyphosis. Fixation and fusion extended from T3 or T4 at the upper level to L5 at the lower level. Facetectomy was performed prior to placement of the wires, and after the rods were wired in place the lateral elements were decorticated and bone graft was placed lateral to the rods to stimulate fusion. In Group II patients, autogenous bone graft supplemented with allograft was used, whereas allograft alone was used in Group III patients. Controlled hypotension was induced during surgery in all cases. A Hemovac drain was left in the subcutaneous tissue.

These patients were monitored at least overnight in the pediatric intensive care unit, with an indwelling arterial catheter for continuous blood pressure recording as well as for monitoring of arterial blood gases. Patients were maintained in the supine position in a regular hospital bed for the first twenty-four hours to tamponade the wound, were allowed to sit up in bed during the first postoperative day, and were encouraged to sit in a chair on the second postoperative day. Early and aggressive mobilization of these patients was stressed.

RESULTS

Group I

The mean correction of curvatures in the Group I patients was 40 percent, with a mean postoperative curvature of forty-three degrees. The average length of postoperative hospitalization in this group was twenty-eight days, with a range of twenty-one to thirty-three days. One patient developed a pressure sore inside the cast, necessitating cast removal at three months, and an orthoplast TLSO was used for further immobilization. Cast or brace immobilization was continued for six months for all patients, and all patients ultimately achieved a solid fusion.

One patient (I-1) who achieved a solid fusion and was brace-free and sitting full-time died following a fulminant respiratory infection eight months postoperatively. Another patient (I-3) was unable to sit fully upright following the procedure because of generalized discomfort and therefore continued to sit in a reclining wheelchair. He died of respiratory failure at age seventeen, four years postoperatively. The final patient (I-3) is still alive at age twenty-one, six years after surgery. He has severe impairment of respiratory function and a vital capacity of less than 5 percent of predicted, but sits full-time with minimal discomfort. For the past year, he has been in a tank respirator during midday naps and at night. His fusion appears solid on radiographs, and there has been no significant change in his curvature.

Group II

The mean correction of curvatures in these patients was 35 percent, with a mean postoperative curve of fifty-four degrees. The average postoperative pelvic obliquity was sixteen degrees, representing a 40 percent correction. In two of these patients (II-1, II-2) prolonged intubation followed by tracheostomy was required for ventilatory support and pulmonary toilet. One of these patients was weaned from the tracheostomy by the fifth postoperative week; however, the other has retained the tracheostomy. Premature extubation of these patients, who had preoperative vital capacities of 30 percent of predicted, may have contributed to their postoperative pulmonary problems. The one patient (II-3) who did not require prolonged ventilatory support stayed in the hospital eighteen days following surgery, while the two who required ventilatory support were hospitalized for forty-nine and fifty-one days.

One patient (II-1) in whom iliac crest bone was taken through the midline incision developed a large subcutaneous hematoma that drained, became infected, and had to be opened to the fascia, which was intact. This wound was treated with dressing changes and subsequently closed spontaneously. This patient also sustained fractures through the osteoporotic bone of his distal tibia and fibula and through the proximal humerus during the postoperative mobilization period.

Two of these patients (II-1 and II-3), at three-and-a-half and four years of follow-up, respectively, are still sitting comfortably full-time. Of these patients, one's curvature is unchanged and the other has increased eight degrees as compared to the six-week postoperative measurement. The third patient (I-2) was sitting comfortably when seen at a six-month postoperative visit; however, he failed to keep further appointments and died approximately three years after surgery. Preoperatively, this patient had the most severe curvature (ninety-six degrees) and following surgery his upper spine remained out of balance. This had worsened by his six-month postoperative visit, leading to concern that head control and sitting balance would become a problem as his muscle weakness progressed.

Group III

The mean curvature correction in these patients was 60 percent, with a mean postoperative curvature of seventeen degrees. The average postoperative pelvic obliquity in the three of five patients for whom both pre- and postoperative measurements were available was two degrees, which represented a 75 percent correction of the pelvic obliquity. All patients were felt to be well balanced postoperatively. Because these curves were relatively mild and still flexible at the time of surgery, bending of the rods to accommodate any residual scoliosis was not necessary, and balance was easily achieved. Rods were contoured to maintain thoracic kyphosis and lumbar lordosis. All patients were extubated the same day as the surgery, and the interval from surgery to discharge for all patients was eight days.

None of these patients experienced any serious immediate postoperative complications, and all were back in school within two weeks of their return home. Two patients (III-3, III-5) experienced left thigh pain, which cleared by the fourth postoperative week. Patient III-4 was readmitted four weeks postoperatively with abdominal pain that was relieved following treatment of a large fecal impaction. Patient III-1 was dropped while being lifted from his wheelchair six weeks after surgery and sustained bilateral supracondylar femur fractures that were treated elsewhere in long leg casts and healed without incident. He continued to sit and showed no evidence of damage to the spine or spinal instrumentation from this fall. The one patient (III-3) who, before surgery, was able to stand in long leg braces has retained this ability for one year postoperatively. For the three patients followed for more than a year since fusion, comparison of their six-week postoperative radiographs and their most recent radiographs shows no significant change in the magnitude of curvature. All of these patients appear to have developed excellent fusion masses.

Because of their rapid mobilization and lack of complications, the patients in this group did not encounter the problems of fatigability and loss of function that are secondary to enforced bed rest. The most notable characteristic of the patients in this group was their rapid return to a normal life style and absence of perioperative complications.

DISCUSSION

It has become relatively well accepted that surgical stabilization of the collapsing spine in patients with Duchenne dystrophy is an appropriate and necessary part of their treatment program (Bunch 1974; Gibson et al. 1978; Renshaw 1982; Robin 1977; Sakai et al. 1977; Swank, Brown, and Perry 1982; Weimann et al. 1983). Patients who have stable, well-balanced spines are able to continue sitting comfortably and have a far better quality of life than those with severe spinal deformities.

Although Harrington instrumentation has proved efficacious for the treatment of spinal deformity, there are disadvantages in the use of this technique for patients with Duchenne muscular dystrophy. The strength of these patients' osteopenic bone at the hook attachment sites is poor, so that both careful handling of patients and external immobilization are required during the postoperative period. A partial solution to this problem may be the use of multiple rods to increase the points of fixation in order to reduce the risk of hook cutout (Bunch 1974). Other disadvantages of the Harrington system are loss of thoracic kyphosis and lumbar lordosis and increased anterior tilt of the pelvis. Reduction of thoracic kyphosis will diminish vital capacity as well as put the patient's head posterior to the center of gravity. By the time most Duchenne muscular dystrophy patients require spinal fusion, they have lost function in their neck flexors. They keep the head forward and use neck extensors against gravity to control the head. If the head is thrown backward, which occurs with straightening of the thoracic kyphosis, this causes loss or impairment of independent head control.

Segmental spinal instrumentation allows the contouring of rods to control sagittal plane alignment in order to retain thoracic kyphosis and lumbar lordosis. Because of the firm fixation it affords, segmental spinal instrumentation also allows rapid mobilization of the patient without the need for a cast or body jacket. Rapid mobilization diminishes the fatiguing effect of surgery, as demonstrated by the fact that the Group III patients required hospitalization for only eight days after surgery and returned to school within two weeks of surgery. The surgery caused minimal interruption in their lives.

The advantage of firm internal stabilization was also demonstrated by the two Group II patients who had significant postoperative pulmonary problems. Although these patients required prolonged mechanical ventilation, repeated bronchoscopy, and aggressive chest physical therapy to treat atelectasis, there was no failure of instrumentation during the handling of these patients. Moreover, in spite of their pulmonary problems, these patients were sitting on the second to third postoperative day. This ability to mobilize them undoubtedly contributed to their survival.

Review of this series of cases indicates that surgery on patients with Duchenne muscular dystrophy at a younger age and with milder curvatures has significant advantages, similar to those observed in patients with spinal muscular atrophy (Riddick, Winter, and Luffer 1982). Pulmonary function in these younger patients is better, their recovery is rapid, and the complication risk is reduced. Correction of curvatures and pelvic obliquity is improved, and balance can be achieved with relative ease when less deformity is present prior to surgery.

Although recommendation of L5 instead of the pelvis as the lower level of instrumentation and fusion awaits confirmation by long-term follow-up in a large group of patients, limited follow-up indicates that this approach is successful on a short-term basis in patients with these milder curvatures, in whom excellent correction and balance can be achieved. The exuberant fusion masses seen in this group of patients may be a result of the combination of the firm fixation plus axial loading, which occurs with segmental instrumentation.

Current information regarding nonoperative control of scoliosis in Duchenne muscular dystrophy indicates that orthoses may delay but cannot prevent the progression of curvature (Hsu 1983). Therefore, if orthoses are used, curvatures will reach the point at which surgery is needed when patients are older and their ability to tolerate these major operations is reduced because of diminution of pulmonary function and decrease in general body strength. Therefore, I currently do not prescribe spinal orthoses for patients with Duchenne muscular dystrophy unless a patient and his family do not wish him to have surgical treatment. For those who will ultimately use surgery as a treatment option, I feel that it is advantageous not to delay curvature progression with a brace and to offer surgical treatment as soon as the untreated curve reaches thirty degrees. Using this approach, patients who develop scoliosis can be treated definitively with segmental spinal instrumentation and fusion at a time when they are better able to tolerate surgery, thereby minimizing risks and maximizing deformity correction and balance of the spine.

REFERENCES

Allen, B. L. and R. L. Ferguson. 1982. "The Galveston Technique for L-Rod Instrumentation of the Scoliotic Spine." *Spine* 7:276-284.

Bunch, W. H. 1974. "Muscular Dystrophy." In J. Hardy, ed. *Spinal Deformity in Neurological and Muscular Disorders*. St. Louis, MO: C. V. Mosby, pp. 2-110.

Gibson, D. A., J. Koreska, D. Robertson, A. Kahn III, and A. M. Albisser. 1978. "The Management of Spinal Deformity in Duchenne's Muscular Dystrophy." *Orthopedic Clinics of North America* 9:437-450.

Herring, J. A. and D. W. Wenger. 1982. "Segmental Spinal Instrumentation." *Spine* 7:285-298.

Hsu, J. D. 1983. "The Natural History of Spine Curvature Progression in the Non-Ambulatory Duchenne Muscular Dystrophy Patient." *Spine* 8:771a-775.

Hsu, J. D., V. M. Hall, S. Swank, R. E. Perry, Jr., J. C. Brown, I. S. Gilgoff, and M. Rapp. 1982. "Control of Spine Curvature in the Duchenne Muscular Dystrophy (DMD) Patient." *Proceedings of the Scoliosis Research Society*, Denver, CO: p. 108.

Johnson, E. W. and S. K. Yarness. 1976. "Hand Dominance and Scoliosis in Duchenne Muscular Dystrophy." *Archives of Physical Medicine and Rehabilitation* 57:462-464.

Kurz, L. T., S. J. Mubarack, P. Schultz, S. M. Park, and J. Leach. 1983. "Correlation of Scoliosis in Pulmonary Function in Duchenne Muscular Dystrophy." *Journal of Pediatric Orthopedics* 3:347-353.

Luque, E. R. and A. Cardoso. 1976. "Segmental Correction of Scoliosis with Rigid Internal Fixation." *Proceedings of the Scoliosis Research Society*, Ottawa, Canada: p. 31.

Luque, E. R. 1982. "The Anatomic Basis and Development of Segmental Spinal Instrumentation." *Spine* 7:256-259.

Renshaw, T. S. 1982. "Treatment of Duchenne's Muscular Dystrophy." *Journal of the American Medical Association* 248:922-923.

Riddick, M. F., R. B. Winter, and L. D. Lutter. 1982. "Spinal Deformities in Patients with Spinal Muscular Atrophy." *Spine* 7:476-483.

Robin, G. C. 1977. "Scoliosis in Duchenne Muscular Dystrophy." *Israel Journal of Medical Science* 13:203-206.

Sakai, D. N., J. D. Hsu, D. A. Bonnett, and J. C. Brown. 1977. "Stabilization of Collapsing Spine in Duchenne Muscular Dystrophy." *Clinical Orthopedics and Related Research* 128:256-260.

Seigel, I. M. 1977. "Orthopedic Correction of Musculoskeletal Deformities in Muscular Dystrophy." *Advances in Neurology* 17:343-364.

Sullivan, J. A. and S. B. Conner. 1982. "Comparison of Harrington Instrumentation and Segmental Spinal Instrumentation in the Management of Neuromuscular Spine Deformities." *Spine* 7:299-304.

Swank, S. M., J. C. Brown, and R. E. Perry. 1982. "Spinal Fusion in Duchenne's Muscular Dystrophy." *Spine* 7:484-491.

Taddonio, R. F. 1982. "Segmental Spinal Instrumentation in the Management of Neuromuscular Spinal Deformity." *Spine* 7:305-311.

Weimann, R. L., D. A. Gibson, C. F. Moseley, and D. C. Jones. 1983. "Surgical Stabilization of the Spine in Duchenne Muscular Dystrophy." *Spine* 8:776-780.

Psychosocial Aspects of Chemotherapy

Anneliese L. Sitarz

Cancer is probably the most feared diagnosis for anyone at any stage of life. When that diagnosis is made in a child, the impact on the whole family and on the treatment team itself is especially intense. The fear of disfigurement is great in both older patients and their families, but it is especially intense in adolescents, who are already struggling with body image.

Parents often express a sense of failure or even shame when their child is diagnosed as having cancer. If the effect of the cancer is not too easily visible and the child's appearance is not altered too much, the parents can usually manage to cope and can help other family members to do so. Any physical changes magnify the problem, however. Transient loss of hair, even when anticipated, is a shock. The weight gain that accompanies treatment with corticosteroids is difficult for many parents. The potential or actual loss of a limb is particularly devastating. Amputation leads not only to the loss of a limb but to the destruction of the whole body image.

If physicians are to be optimally effective in treating children with cancer, they must, in fact, be family practitioners and must familiarize themselves with the psychodynamics in their patients' immediate and extended families. Yet they must not be so involved that they lose objectivity with respect to the treatment. This is not easy. Treatment must be selected in terms of curing the cancer, but the potential long-term effects of that treatment on the growing child must also be kept in mind. Now that many cancers are curable and the number of survivors is increasing, the late effects of treat-

Anneliese L. Sitarz, MD, is Professor of Clinical Pediatrics, Department of Pediatrics, College of Physicians and Surgeons, Columbia University, New York, NY.

© 1988 by The Haworth Press, Inc. All rights reserved.

ment, even secondary malignancies, are being observed. Although it must be realized that a person who gets one cancer may be more prone to get another, it is an inescapable possibility that some treatment modalities may increase the likelihood that the patient will develop another malignancy. Thus, it becomes increasingly imperative to tailor treatment as much as possible to the specific cancer type and also to the stage and potential severity of the disease. The treatment must be aggressive, yet the risk of toxicity or long-term side effects must be kept as low as possible.

In order to achieve this balance, patients are often randomly assigned to different arms of a treatment protocol. When this approach is explained to parents who must make a decision about the treatment plan for their child, and to the older patient, the parents and the patient are caught between fear of the cancer and fear of being used as a "guinea pig." It is up to the physician to explain in detail why a particular treatment is recommended or why random assignment is being done. For the average parent, this means confronting extremely difficult decisions at a time when they are reeling from the shock of the diagnosis. In fact, they are asked to sign so-called informed consent forms before the treatment can begin. Whether this consent is ever really "informed" is an open question.

The physician must be able to recognize and deal with the parents' emotional distress in this dilemma in a way that will enable them to make a meaningful decision. An explanation of the results of previous protocols that have led to improved survival over the years may be helpful. Assurance must also be given that a treatment program will be stopped or changed if the anticipated results are not attained or if serious adverse reactions occur. Although a reasonable effort must be made to explain the potential side effects, care must be taken to put the risks and benefits into proper perspective, lest the parents get the feeling that the treatment is worse than the disease.

It is usually helpful to discuss the diagnosis and treatment plans with the parents in the presence of the social worker and the pediatric psychiatric nurse or to have these members of the treatment team meet with the parents and child shortly afterward to lend necessary support. This is useful because parents often have difficulty comprehending all that is being said to them in this stressful period.

Enlisting various members of the treatment team ensures that there are other people who have heard the discussion and can reinforce its important aspects later.

It has frequently been said in parent group sessions that the parents did not fully understand the often lengthy consent forms that they were given to sign before the child's treatment could be started. Many parents feel that they really have no choice and want to sign without reading the material. Getting them to read the consent form and to understand the treatment rationale serves more than a legal purpose. Because the parents know their child best, they are an important part of the treatment team, and therefore need as much information as possible to be able to carry through with the needed treatments. Also, the more they understand, the less helpless they feel — and standing by, unable to help, is probably one of the hardest things to bear. Some parents are too numb at first to understand how they will help, but when they do, it helps them to cope with the situation. The better the parents cope, the better the child will cope and tolerate the treatments.

Once the parents have accepted the diagnosis and the treatment plan, these must be explained to the child. What the child is told and in how much detail obviously depends on the child's age. While older teenagers should usually be included in the treatment decision-making process, even young children need to have some understanding of the chronicity of the disease and the treatment, as well as the need for certain procedures or treatments. This understanding will help them to cope more readily with the attendant discomforts or side effects and with their necessary duration. The latter is especially difficult for younger patients to comprehend, since time has a different meaning for them than for adults. In addition, learning to take medicine regularly, and especially to swallow pills, may be difficult for them. Practicing with TicTacs or M&Ms may be useful; disguising medication in honey, chocolate syrup, jam, or applesauce can also help.

Many chemotherapeutic agents cause nausea or vomiting. Hair loss, bleeding, jaw and leg pains, obesity, increased susceptibility to infection, and liver, kidney, or heart damage can occur. When the child is symptomatic from the disease, these complications of treatment are more readily tolerated. When improvement has occurred and the child feels well, the need to continue chemotherapy can be more difficult to accept. When treatment involves parenteral medication, the pain of injection is added to other possible side effects. No matter how small the needle, it remains a needle to the child and is feared. Necessary restraint adds to the fearfulness. Yet even very young children adapt amazingly quickly and recognize when something will hurt and when not. Many three-year-olds will hold out their hand for a Vincristine injection with barely a wince once they are familiar with the procedure. It is important that it be made clear to the child from the start that the treatment is not a form of punishment for some wrong. Similarly, parents should be warned that the threat of an injection should never be used in a disciplinary manner.

For older children or teenagers, the need to comply with a medical regimen holds an additional threat: the loss of independence just at a time when they covet increased independence. Not only is the treatment schedule limiting, but many of the drug side effects are too. Nausea and vomiting are debilitating. Hair loss, a Chushingoid body, the need to stay away from others when the white count is low, the threat of bleeding when there is thrombocytopenia—all of these effects are devastating. The inability for children to go to school and to be in the mainstream of life for their age group can be severely depressing. When they become bald or develop marked obesity, some children withdraw from their peers. Others adapt by regressing to more immature, dependent roles. Some are very angry—in either an overt or covert manner—and may express their anger by refusing to take further medication in any form. This, naturally, is deeply distressing to the parents, who themselves are torn between fear of the drugs and the knowledge that the child will die without them. In such situations, physicians and parents are confronted by the dilemma of having to convince children of the importance of continuing to take medication without frightening them more than necessary about the disease. They need to recognize that children's anger results from increased frustration. Hypnosis and psychotherapy have been used successfully in dealing with such patients.

How much of a burden chemotherapy can be for children is shown most clearly in some patients whose treatment has been completed. An increasing number of childhood patients are surviving now, and many parents report a real personality change in such children when they no longer face the repetitive need to take medication, even when this was given only by mouth. These children appear freer and happier than before and their schoolwork seems to improve. These changes, which appear to be as much psychological as physical, are seen even in very young patients and even in patients who had no obvious problems with side effects.

For the parents, the mechanics of a chemotherapeutic regimen also require adjustment. Not only does chemotherapy have to be given regularly on a predetermined schedule, but in many instances it is given in the hospital or outpatient clinic and requires many hours or days there, which disrupts family routine. The idea that strong, potentially toxic chemicals are given to their children creates powerful emotional conflicts. Quite a few parents question the use of chemotherapy for fear the child will be maimed or "poisoned" by it. If the tumor has been excised or amputated, they may question the need for further treatment, or they may recognize the need but fear the drugs. Having the parents of newly diagnosed children meet families who are further along in the treatment program is often helpful. When they can see another child apparently tolerating the same or similar treatment well, it becomes more tolerable for them too.

In attempting to obtain a family's acceptance of a given treatment program, the interactions of the extended family—that is, siblings, grandparents, and aunts and uncles—need to be considered. Occasionally, the relatives try to undermine the treatment by questioning whether the child really has cancer or by suggesting some other treatment, sometimes of questionable value. One grandfather, who insisted that the doctors were poisoning his granddaughter, was deeply disturbed when, in addition, the radiotherapy ports were outlined on her head—"marking up" his granddaughter, as he put it. His attitude was distressing to the child's mother, his daughter, who was divorced and had had to make all of the decisions herself. In dealing with such problems, it sometimes helps to suggest to parents that the other family members be included in meetings with the physician at which the diagnosis or the potential treatment course is discussed. The more thoroughly all of the family members understand what is going on, the more they can support each other. Despite such meetings, even parents who appear to be quite sophisticated may at times turn from what they consider to be "toxic" treatment to such forms of treatment as food fads, megavitamins, or unproven agents recommended by someone at home. These families may test the patience of the medical personnel, especially when the child has what can now be considered a curable cancer and is denied treatment that is known to be effective. Every effort must be made to explain the true situation to the parents and perhaps to enlist the help of a close friend or member of the clergy. If these efforts fail to convince the parents to allow proper treatment, it may be necessary to obtain a court order to enable treatment to continue. The child's life and welfare must come first and must be protected to the extent allowed by law until the child is old enough to make decisions for himself or herself.

A significant factor in giving chemotherapy is the cost of some of the drugs. A single treatment course can cost hundreds of dollars. For young families, this creates a tremendous financial burden. Yet there are sources of financial help, and it is important to identify these sources for the parents. This is where well-informed social workers can be extremely helpful. They can suggest or even mediate contact with the Leukemia Society of America, the Cancer Society, or individually supported foundations that help to defray the cost of cancer treatment.

The doctors and nurses caring for these children must not only explain the diagnosis and treatments in terms that are understandable to the parents and the children, they must also acquire the expertise to make the treatment as free of discomfort as possible. Finding veins in order to give intravenous chemotherapy to chubby, squirming toddlers can be difficult. The need to give painful treatments such as bone marrow aspirations, spinal taps, or intravenous medications is not without trauma for the medical staff either. It is not easy to have to be the person who inflicts pain, especially when this is repetitive and the patient is too young to understand why this is happening.

With patients who are younger than age three, it is probably best to do what has to be done as quickly as possible, with gentle restraint as needed, and without lengthy discussion. At about that age, however, time spent in gaining the child's cooperation and confidence pays untold dividends. Even at this young age, a child can, after a relatively short time, understand the need to hold still and realize the brevity of the pain, and may then require little or no restraint. The promise of a Band-aid, which has an almost magical connotation to a child insofar as it signifies the end of the painful procedure, or a lollipop, can enhance cooperation.

As indicated earlier, it is a bit easier to explain why a given treatment is necessary when the patient is sick or in pain. However, older children have difficulty accepting painful procedures or taking medications that may make them feel sick when, without the medications, they actually feel well.

Children frequently express anger at the nurse or physician involved. Unless this anger is understood and dealt with appropriately, it makes the treatment period more difficult, not only for the child and the staff involved, but also for the parents. The parents may be torn between empathy with the child's feelings and a degree of embarrassment toward the staff. They need guidance in helping the child express anger in acceptable ways; that is, the child can cry, but hitting or biting should be reprimanded. Some people think that it helps children when they are told that they can scream as loudly as they want when something hurts as long as they do not move. I have always questioned this, since it encourages further loss of control for children who already feel helpless in the face of all they must endure. I have always told children that it is all right to cry, but that screaming is unnecessary. I try to outline what I am doing as I go along and to stick to a given ritual for each procedure in order to reduce children's fear of the unknown. I refuse to shout above their screams. I say that if they want to hear what I am saying, they must not make too much noise. This usually has a calming effect and the children require less restraint.

On occasion, one must deal with uncontrollable anger in the parents as well. Their anger stems from the fear aroused by the diagnosis and the frustration of having to go through a lengthy and burdensome treatment period. Their anger may be overt and confrontational or it may be expressed as endless complaints about minor problems. The anger is vented on the physicians and nurses caring for the child and at times on other parents on the ward, but must be recognized for what it is. In the midst of a hectic day, dealing with such anger creates an additional burden on the staff in its effort to care for a given patient. Especially when the child is *not* doing well, dealing with such anger adds to the frustration the staff feels at not being able to cure the child. This can lead to intense emotional stress. Group meetings with all of those involved can be useful and should be held frequently when such a situation exists. Again, it may be helpful to call on other parents to give much-needed support to the family at such a time.

As much as parents fear the start of chemotherapy, the decision to stop it, for whatever reasons, can also be difficult and stressful. Some parents have stated at group meetings that the day that chemotherapy was to be stopped, after their child had been given treatment for the required course and appeared to be free of disease, was second only to the day they first heard the diagnosis in terms of the stress created. As much as parents look forward to the end of the treatment period, the once-feared medications assume the role of a crutch; their fear that the disease could recur if the drugs are no longer given is intense.

However, an even more emotionally charged issue is the decision to cease treatment because the patient is no longer responding. Although parents should not be asked to make a decision that may be difficult for them to live with after the child has died, their underlying concerns, fears, wishes, and emotions must be an important part of the decision-making process. Most parents feel a sense of guilt concerning the child's illness, and this should not be reinforced by asking them to make a decision about stopping treatment. On the other hand, if the child has been suffering, the parents may have wished to have the treatment stopped, and may be relieved if the suggestion to cease chemotherapy comes from someone else, so long as they are assured that every effort will be made to keep the child comfortable. Some parents may insist on a given course of action, such as no further treatment, only to reverse that decision a short while later. For example, on one afternoon, one mother was adamant in her determination that, in order to spare her son further pain, he be given no further chemotherapy. Two hours later, however, she called the physician to ask that everything possible still be done for her son. At such times, parents may actually express gratitude to the physician who assures them that they will not have to make such a decision alone. The staff must remain keenly sensitive to the family's feelings and intermittent ambivalence at these times.

Insofar as possible, older children should be included in any considerations regarding the termination of treatment. At times they may say that they do not want any more treatment and yet, a short while later, express the fear that the physician might stop the treatment, thus indicating or confirming the hopelessness of their situation. Nevertheless, these patients will often verbalize their wishes, fears, and concerns. Frequently, older children will confide their real wishes to a trusted nurse while avoiding the issue with their parents in an attempt to protect them. Even some young children have an amazing insight into their parents' concerns and will use rather elaborate means to protect them or even try to comfort them if they appear to be sad or upset. I have, for example, seen a three-year-old take her mother's hand to comfort her when she saw her mother cry. There may be extensive "mutual protection" in some families, with the result that true communication is nearly impossible. In such situations, members of the staff may be able to intervene and mediate better communication to prevent the resulting isolation of the patient.

It must be recognized that the need to deal with all of these issues with both the family and the patient can be emotionally draining for the staff. Although many physicians find this work rewarding, some simply cannot cope with these patients; others do so by becoming increasingly task-oriented, and still others delegate the interaction to someone else, retaining only a supervisory stance themselves. The current trend toward group care of these patients is partly an attempt to lessen the stresses. Although reducing involvement with patient diminishes the stress on the staff, the patient is denied the close physician-patient relationship that is so important in this type of chronic illness.

Those staff members who do deal effectively with patients need to be able to compensate for the stress in some way. They must learn to "leave the problems at the hospital" and must cultivate absorbing hobbies in their limited free time or manage to get away frequently for short vacations. Although much progress in patients' survival has been made in the last few years, much more still needs to be accomplished, and caring for these patients will continue to challenge the physical and emotional resources of everyone involved. Emotional exhaustion, or burnout, can become a reality and can make it impossible for staff members to function in the most productive manner.

The Ultimate Loss:
The Dying Child

Dottie C. Wilson

The concept of hospice or palliative care is familiar to most health care professionals today, and to a large segment of the general population. It has been welcomed enthusiastically as an alternative for the care of terminally ill patients. When aggressive therapy for cure or the prolongation of life is no longer appropriate, or when the distressing side effects outweigh the benefits of acute treatment, then the emphasis shifts to a palliative care or hospice approach. In this approach, the focus is on the quality rather than the quantity of the remaining life. This approach emphasizes the management of pain and other distressing symptoms and treatment of both the whole person and the person's family by addressing their psychosocial, emotional, spiritual, and economic needs. An interdisciplinary team approach to care is essential in addressing these multifaceted needs.

Hospice or palliative care for terminally ill children is not yet a familiar concept. Such care recognizes that dying children and their families can benefit equally from this approach: pediatric palliative care requires equal attention to pain and symptom management and to medical and nursing care, as well as emphasis on family support, home care, and day care, with specialized inpatient backup. Because this is a relatively new and untried approach, special attention must be given to research, evaluation, and education (Wilson 1982). It has been found that the needs of dying children and their families and the ways to meet these needs are similar, but not identical, to those of dying adults and their families (Wilson 1985).

Dottie C. Wilson is affiliated with the Palliative Care Center, St. Mary's Hospital for Children, Bayside, NY.

© 1988 by The Haworth Press, Inc. All rights reserved.

In most communities, dying children form only a small group of patients. This is indeed fortunate, except for the fact that programs exclusively for these children are difficult to establish and to support financially. This, along with the tendency to treat children aggressively to the end, may help explain why there are so few programs especially designed for terminally ill children. As compared to adult patients, the population of patients ranging in the age from birth to about eighteen years is characterized by greater variations in physical size, developmental levels, medical conditions, and handicaps, as well as greater diversity of interests and communication abilities. Also, the diversity of diagnoses among terminally ill children requires special services and skills, whereas in adult programs there is at present but one major diagnosis—cancer.

The families of these patients tend to be much larger in number than the families of patients in adult programs and frequently include not only parents and siblings but also grandparents, aunts and uncles, and school and neighborhood friends. Usually, at least the younger family members have not faced a death before. The loss is felt more strongly by all concerned when it is a child who dies. Families—particularly parents—are accustomed to caring for their children and making decisions for them. There may be conflicts among the wishes of the parents, the child, and the staff, and these may present unexpected difficulties. The more the family is involved in the child's care, the more they benefit later in that their sense of guilt when the child dies tends to be less, reducing their anguish. This finding is confirmed by Martinson's studies (1979).

To care for these children in a special hospice or palliative care program, special attention to selection, training, and support of staff is essential. To meet the wide-ranging needs of this population of patients, staff members need to be particularly sensitive, have diversified medical and psychosocial knowledge and skills, and feel comfortable supporting both children and adults. When such staff members can be found and are able to work together as an interdisciplinary team, they can meet the challenges of caring for these patients and their families and thereby gain the satisfaction of making an important contribution.

St. Mary's Hospital for Children has developed a unique program, the Palliative Care Center, to provide this care. The center, which, because of the special situations involving children, has not applied for state certification as a hospice, opened in October 1984. It is the culmination of the hospital's commitment over the past six years to the development of a full-scale pediatric terminal care program, including home care, day care, inpatient care, and bereavement care, as well as research and educational functions. St. Mary's Hospital is a skilled nursing facility. It was founded in 1870 and is still owned and operated by the Sisters of St. Mary, a religious order of the Episcopal Church.

Since there is little experience at this time in specialized pediatric terminal care programs, the Palliative Care Center is breaking new ground in many aspects of its work. Home care is provided by the hospital's Long Term Home Health Care Program, the only one of its kind specializing in the care of children in the state. The ten-bed inpatient unit is the first of its kind in this country to be specifically designed, equipped, and staffed for terminally ill children of different ages and having different diagnoses, abilities, and interests, and for their families. In a noninstitutional, park-like setting overlooking Little Neck Bay and its boats, the unit includes large activity areas, terraces, skylights, large windows, and family spaces, as well as carefully designed and equipped patient rooms and nursing work areas. Family members of all ages may visit at any time, enjoy meals there, and, when needed, sleep overnight next to the patient's bed. The atmosphere is that of a warm, loving, caring community.

The children accepted at the center are those sixteen years of age or younger who have a life expectancy of one year or less, who need palliative care services, and whose family and physician agree to the admission. The diagnoses that are considered appropriate include not only cancer but also end-stage cardiac disease; degenerative neurological, pulmonary, and renal diseases; and end-stage orthopedic problems.

The center's four major goals are defined as follows:

1. To provide expert interdisciplinary team care for the management of pain and other distress.
2. To meet the needs and wishes of each patient and family and to

help them experience new awareness and meaning in their lives.

3. To assist both the patient and family in their understanding of the patient's condition and to support them during this stressful time.

4. To continue supporting the family after the child's death.

Family support is an extremely important part of pediatric palliative care. In the center, families who are receiving home care, day care, and inpatient services are encouraged to express their fears, anger, guilt, and grief, and are helped to deal with these feelings.

Families suffer the death of a child more severely than that of an adult. Fischoff and O'Brien (1976) have pointed out that "the parents feel the loss of their child as if they have lost a part of themselves, which, indeed, they have." Major problems may arise between the two parents, since the child's death strikes both of them simultaneously. As Rando (1985) has noted, because both parents are grieving deeply, neither partner is able to rely fully on the other as a therapeutic resource and, indeed, the closeness of marriage makes it likely that partners will displace their feelings of anger and blame onto each other.

Siblings, too, suffer not only the loss of the child but may also feel the loss of their own security. Will they also die? Will their parents be unable to protect them, too? All members of the extended family — grandparents, other relatives, and friends — suffer from the death. The accepted order of things, that older people die before younger people, is shattered, leaving those who loved the child confused and shaken. Reorganizing the family system to function without the child is part of the family's grief work (Arnold and Gemma 1983).

The length of bereavement following the death of a child is longer than that following the death of an adult. Whereas in adult programs families are usually followed for a year after the death, Corr, Martinson, and Dyer (1985) found that more than 20 percent of families in their study reported that their most intense grief had not ended at twenty-four months after the child's death. For another 25 percent, the most intense grief lasted for twelve to eighteen months after the child's death. It also seems clear that sibling bereavement continues even longer than that of parents.

To meet the needs of those suffering the loss of a child, the Palliative Care Center's bereavement care program provides ongoing support to families for as long as needed, with the length of time expected to be from one to three years. Since the program is so new, experiential data are not yet available. Families are followed through home visits, phone calls, school visits, and support groups by specially trained volunteers who are supervised by an experienced bereavement coordinator. Weekly bereavement team meetings are held to review cases and, with the assistance of a psychiatrist or psychologist, to identify those suffering abnormal grief and arrange professional help for them. Staff members who are grieving over the loss of a child they have cared for are also supported by individual and group sessions and memorial services.

Through the bereavement care program and a consistently caring approach throughout the center, staff and volunteers affirm the legitimacy of the grief that family members feel, encourage them to proceed through their grief work, comfort them, and give hope for relief from their pain with time. Active listening and encouraging the continuing reiteration of events and feelings are helpful. So is just being present and demonstrating empathetic caring. Thus, through time, families can complete the process of coming to terms with loss, can resolve their concerns about the reasons for and meaning of the event, can learn to cope without the child, and can achieve a reintegration of their lives. The loss is never forgotten but, with help, the emotional ties are released.

REFERENCES

Arnold, J. H. and P. B. Gemma. 1983. *A Child Dies: A Portrait of Family Grief.* Rockville, MD: Aspen Systems Corporation.

Corr, C. A., I. M. Martinson, and K. L. Dyer. 1985. "Parental Bereavement." In C. A. Corr and D. M. Corr, eds. *Hospice Approaches to Pediatric Care.* New York: Springer Publishing Co.

Fischoff, J. and N. O'Brien. 1976. "After the Child Dies." *Journal of Pediatrics* 88:140-146.

Martinson, I. M. 1979. "Caring for the Dying Child." *Nursing Clinics of North America* 14:467-474.

Rando, A. 1985. *Grief, Dying, and Death: Clinical Interventions for Caregivers*. Champaign, IL: Research Press Co.

Wilson, D. C. 1982. "The Viability of Pediatric Hospices: A Case Study." *Death Education* 6:205-212.

Wilson, D. C. 1985. "Developing a Hospice Program for Children." In C. A. Corr and D. M. Corr, eds. *Hospice Approaches to Pediatric Care*. New York: Springer Publishing Co.

Communication Among Children, Parents, and Funeral Directors

Daniel J. Schaefer

I have been a funeral director for the last twenty-five years. My family has been in the funeral service for one hundred and seven years. We have buried our friends; I have buried parents of my friends and children of my friends. Over the last ten years or so, I have found that something is missing: there have been fewer children attending funerals than I knew were in my friends' families. I began to ask parents, very simply, "What are you saying to your kids about this death in your family?" The replies of 1,800 sets of the parents of more than 3,600 children proved that they were basically unprepared to talk with their children about death and terribly uneasy about doing so, but not unwilling to say something once they were prepared by someone or given appropriate information.

The bits of information that I am going to present are not a standard message. They are building materials. The blueprint is individual to each family, so what we do is to take the family's blueprint, which has their particular death circumstance, then take the building materials, and build a message that parents can give to their

Daniel J. Schaefer is a funeral director, Brooklyn, NY.

© 1988 by The Haworth Press, Inc. All rights reserved.

children. For the families that I serve, I do this on an individual basis.

TALKING TO CHILDREN ABOUT DEATH

Thinking about talking to children about death is upsetting. It makes many parents anxious. It has been helpful for parents to know how many other parents feel. On Memorial Day two years ago, at three in the morning, I received a call that my brother had been killed in an automobile accident. I have five children, and I knew that four hours from then I was going to have to explain to them about their uncle. I said to my wife, "It's unusual — I've done this with hundreds of families, but I have this thing in the pit of my stomach. I *know* what to say to these kids; I know exactly what I'm going to do. Can you imagine how it must be for somebody who doesn't know what to say?"

What do people say about speaking to children about death? Some are sure that they do have to talk to their children and some say they are not sure that it is necessary. Some parents who believe that something should be said are told by others that they should avoid upsetting their children. Parents naturally tend to build a protective wall around their children. What I say to them is "Let's look at the wall, let's see if it works, and if it does work, who is it working for? Is it working for you, to protect you from your child's grief? If we look over the wall, what do we see on the other side? Do we see a kid who is comfortable or do we see, in fact, a kid who is a solitary mourner?"

When parents plan to speak to their children about death, they have to understand that what they are about to do is not easy, that they are going to be upset and stressed, that they are probably going to lack energy, and that they are going to feel unable to concentrate. They are going to be afraid of their own emotions and the effect that these emotions will have on their children. They are not going to know what their children understand, and basically they have to realize that they want to protect their children from pain. It is important that parents know ahead of time that they are going to feel this way.

What do other people say to them? They say, "Your kids don't know what's going on," "Wait until later," "Tell them a fairy tale," "Don't say anything," "Send them away until the funeral is over," or "Do you really want to put your kids through all this?" implying that no loving parent would. It is almost frightening to talk with one's children on this subject, but I believe that it is dangerous not to.

Almost all parents will agree that children are surprisingly perceptive. They overhear conversations, read emotions and responses around them, and ask questions, directly and indirectly. They *will* receive messages; it is impossible not to communicate. No matter how hard parents try not to, they are going to communicate their grief to their children. Without some explanation, the children will be confused and anxious. What I say to parents is, "Since you're going to be sending a message out anyway, why don't you try to control the message?" A message is controlled by making sure that the information is true, geared for the age of the child, and, if possible, delivered in surroundings that make the child's reception of the message a little easier to handle.

For parents, feeling in control is important at a time when feeling out of control is routine and common, and when helping the child — the most dependent person in the family at that time — is also critical. The discussion between parent and child may be the child's only chance to understand what is happening. Sometimes, however, the pressure and enormity of this task, along with the advice of others, really proves too great for parents. They choose a short-term covering for themselves, without realizing the long-term effect on their children.

Explaining the How and Why of Death

Children have to know from the beginning what sad is. They have to know why their parents are sad and why they themselves are sad. So parents can begin with, "This is a very sad time," or "A very sad thing has happened," or "Mommy and Daddy are sad because. . . ." Children have to know that it is a death that has made the parents sad: with no explanation, they may think that they have caused the sadness. They also have to know that it is appropriate to feel sad.

The next stage involves an explanation of death and what it means. Death basically means that a person's body stops working and will not work any more. It won't do any of the things it used to do. It won't walk, talk, or move; none of its parts work; it does not see and it does not hear. This foundation is what parents feel comfortable referring back to when children ask questions like "Will Grandpa ever move again?" "Why can't they fix him?" "Why isn't he moving?" "Is he sleeping?" "Can he hear me?" "Can he eat after he's buried?" If parents come up with different answers to all of these questions, it becomes confusing, but when they have a foundation, they can come back to it repeatedly. The notion that something has stopped working is a firm foundation for children, and parents feel comfortable in not lying or deceiving in using this type of explanation.

Because death is a form of abandonment, the words "passed away," "gone away," or "left us," that many people use hold out to the child the hope that the deceased will return, which of course causes tremendous frustration while they wait for the person to return. Appropriate explanations to children of why a particular death happened might be, for example, in a case of terminal illness, "Because the disease couldn't be stopped. The person became very, very sick, the body wore out, and the body stopped working"; in a case of suicide, "Some people's bodies get sick and don't work right, and some people's minds don't work right. They can't see things clearly, and they feel that the only way to solve their problems is to take their own life"; in a case of miscarriage, "Sometimes a baby is just starting to grow; something happens and makes it stop. We don't know what it was — it wasn't anything that anyone did."

CHILDREN'S REACTIONS TO DEATH

When people start to take this information and relate it to their own family situations in preparation for confronting their families, they want to know what they need to be concerned about and what to look for. Even newborn infants and toddlers know when things are different. The smaller they are, the less likely it is that they will be able to figure out why. Children respond to changes in behavior;

they sense when life patterns change. Infants may alter their nursing patterns; toddlers become cranky, and change their sleeping and eating patterns. Excitement at home, new people around, parents gone at odd times, a significant person missing, a sad atmosphere — children know that something is different and react accordingly. When parents expect these changes in their children, they can respond to them more sensibly.

Piaget says that children between the ages of three and six years see death as reversible. The way this translates for parents (and for children) is that people will come back, that dead is not forever. Parents have said to me, "How could a child think that somebody will return?" From a child's point of view, ET returns, Jesus and Lazarus returned, and Road Runner returns constantly. And children may misinterpret the rise-again eulogies often given by clergy.

Several years ago (1978), "Sesame Street" produced a program dealing with the death of Mr. Hooper. The program was written up in newspapers and other publications as being an advance for the education of children. The problem is that Mr. Hooper has returned in reruns of the show, so that children who experienced his death now find that Mr. Hooper is back again.

People may say, "My child isn't affected by his grandfather's death — he's only four years old." I say, "Why should he be affected? As far as he's concerned, Grandpa's only going to be dead for a little while." Knowing how children perceive death helps parents to understand their children better, so that they will not become upset when a child continues to ask questions. They know that children in that age range can be expected to ask more questions.

Children also tend to connect events that are not connected. Does this death mean that someone else is going to die? "Grandpa died after he had a headache. Mommy has a headache. Does that mean that she is going to die?" "Old people die. Daddy is old [he is thirty]. Is he going to die?" This means that we have to explain the difference between being very, very sick and just sick like Mommy or Daddy might be; the difference between being very, very old and over twenty; and the difference between being very old and very sick and being very old but not very sick.

Children ages six to nine know that death is final, but they still think about return. They need a more detailed explanation of why a person has died than younger children do. With these children, it is much more important to distinguish between a fatal illness and just being sick—to say, "It's not like when you get sick, or when Mommy or Daddy get sick." If a parent tells a child, "Grandpa had a pain in his stomach, went to the hospital, and died," what is the child to think the next time that Mommy has menstrual cramps? What are children to think when a grandparent dies from lung cancer after a tremendous bout of coughing and then find that their father has a cough? It is normal for children in that situation to start to cling to the father and ask, "Are you okay?"

Children of this age may not want to go to a house where a person has died because "it's spooky." They also have to deal with and understand their emotions, to know that crying, feeling bad, and being angry are all acceptable behaviors.

Children ages nine to twelve move much closer to an adult sense of grieving. They are more aware of the details of an illness and more aware of the impact of a death on them. Consequently, they need more emotional support. They need to know that their feelings are acceptable and that someone is supportive of those feelings.

Teenagers also need support with their new feelings. Parents may find it better to share their own feelings with their adolescent children. Teenagers also have to understand why a person has died.

At the funeral of a friend, I met a man I used to know, another funeral director. He said to me, "It's strange. When I grew up in Queens with my grandfather, we lived in a two-family house for ten-and-a-half years. When my parents had enough money, they bought a house on Long Island, and we moved there. That was in the summer. On my birthday, in October, Grandpa didn't send me a card. I was a little concerned about that, but when Grandpa didn't come for Thanksgiving, and then when he didn't come for Christmas, I asked my mother where Grandpa was. She said he couldn't come." My friend went on: "I couldn't think what I could possibly have done to this dear man that I had spent my childhood with that would cause him not to like me any more. Then it went on again. Grandpa never came in the summer, then it was another Thanksgiving and another Christmas. It wasn't until I was thirteen that they told me that my grandfather had died. I thought that was bizarre until a woman came into my funeral home three weeks ago and when I said to her, as I say to everybody, 'What did you say to your kids about the death of your mother?' she said, 'I haven't told them. I just told them she went on a vacation in Vermont.'" So the difference between ten years ago, or fifteen, or twenty years ago and today is not so great for uninformed parents.

Responsibility

People say, "How can a child feel responsible for the death of another person?" Yet, they will say to their children, "You're driving me crazy," "You'll be the death of me yet," or "Don't give me a heart attack!" Adults may say such things as figures of speech, but children do not always see it that way. "If only I had prayed harder," they may say. Children basically see God as a rewarder or punisher; He rewards good behavior and punishes bad. Therefore, if a child does a bad thing that only he or she knows about, God may punish the child by the death of someone in the child's family. If illness or death follows a misdeed, the child can feel really responsible for this. For example, when a parent leaves the home, a child may say, "If I had cleaned my room (done my chores, hadn't wet my pants, done better in school), maybe he (or she) wouldn't have left." This is what happens when no explanation is given to a child about why a person has died. When a grandparent stops visiting, the child again may say, "What did I do?"

Magical Thinking

Some children believe that by wishing that a person will die, they can cause the person's death. They sometimes also believe that if they think about the death of a person who is dying, they themselves may die.

Anger

This is a common response at the time of a death and one that is extremely damaging to families. Understanding it and anticipating its presence helps families deal with anger from both sides, the parent's and the children's. Children can be angry at parents for not telling them that the deceased was sick, for having spent so much time with the deceased and not enough time with them, for not allowing them to attend the funeral, or just because they need someone to be angry at.

I offer two examples of children's anger at parents. When my brother died, two days after the funeral there was a tremendous downpour. There were two inches of water in the back yard, and my ten-year-old son came to me and said, "I want to pitch my tent in the back yard." I said, "David, you can't pitch a tent. There are two inches of water in the yard!" He became angry, threw the tent down, and walked away. I said to him, "Look, I'll tell you why you're angry: you don't have anyone to be angry at. You can't be angry at your uncle because he was in an automobile accident. He wasn't drunk and he wasn't driving fast. It was a wet road, he didn't know it, and the car turned over and he was killed. You can't be angry at the doctors or the hospital because he was dead when he arrived there." I said, "There's nobody else to be angry at, so the next possibility is to be angry at me. As long as you understand that, it's okay." He came back a while later and said, "You know, after thinking about it, I don't know why I ever wanted to pitch my tent in the yard."

The second example came a few days ago when I spoke to a woman about coming to a funeral. She said, "You know, I was seven years old when they took me to my grandfather's funeral. I could go to the funeral, I could sit outside — my parents even bought me a brand new dress — but I was not allowed to go in and say goodbye to Grandpa. So you know what? I never wore the dress again and I never talked about Grandpa again."

Children can also be angry at themselves for wishing that a person would die or for not visiting or helping a dying person. One young boy had seen his grandfather walking down the street carrying some packages and noticed that his grandfather was not doing so well. But Grandfather did not do well a lot of the time, so the boy helped his grandfather take the packages inside, went on home, and did not say anything to his father about his grandfather. The grandfather died of a heart attack in the house. Later, the boy's father came to me and asked, "What am I going to say? My son said, 'If only I'd told you this time that Grandpa didn't look well, maybe we could have done something.'" Two weeks ago a mother came to me and said, "My daughter thinks that my mother may have died because she failed to send her a get-well card. She thought that maybe it would have saved her if she had sent it."

The driver of a car, the doctor at a hospital, the deceased for putting themselves in dangerous situations, even the event that caused a death—these are just a few examples of the legitimate targets of children's anger. When parents know that children are responding with anger or that they may do so, the parents will do best if they address it directly with the children. The important point for parents is that they feel much more in control when they can anticipate this kind of anger. They know the historical background of their old circumstances, their own blueprint, and if they consider these they can help their children through their anger.

Guilt

This is another aspect of grief and grieving. Knowing that a child may feel guilty, or having it pointed out, lets parents know that their children can, on one hand, be angry at the deceased and, on the other, feel guilty about being angry. Children may express their guilt in statements such as "I didn't do enough," "I should have visited him before he died," and "If only I hadn't gone to the movies last week instead of going to see Grandpa, I would have been able to say goodbye before he died." All of these "shoulds" and "if onlys" can have a tremendous impact on a family if they are not directed, if nobody anticipates them, and if nobody explains them to the children.

CHILDREN AND FUNERALS

People feel the need to know how to explain what is going to happen next: "After I've explained to my children that this person has died, what do I say to them about what's going to happen now?" I have some material in script form that I offer to families, but basically parents have to start from the beginning with a child. They can say, "Grandpa will be taken from where he died to a funeral home; it's a place where they'll keep him for a few days until he's buried. He'll be dressed in clothes he liked and put into a casket—that's a box we use so that no dirt gets on him when he's buried. People will come to the funeral home to visit and say how sorry they are that Grandpa has died. Because his body isn't working any more, it won't move or do any of the things it used to do, but if you want to come and say some prayers, you can.''

The basic premise here is that people will ask whether or not they should bring a child to the funeral home. People are surprised when I say, ''Never! Don't ever bring children to a funeral home if you're not going to prepare them for it ahead of time.'' My son had cardiac surgery a year and a half ago. Before his operation, they showed him the operating room, the recovery room, and the intensive care unit. He knew everything that was going to happen to him before he went into the hospital for the surgery. His doctor even drew a diagram of the operation for him and made a model of the surgical repair out of clay for him. But people will still waltz children into a funeral home and say, ''We're just going to see Grandma.'' Then they wonder why the children are upset when they walk in and find out that Grandma is lying down in a casket and not moving.

Children should be treated like people and given the same concern we give anyone else. They should hear an explanation of what will happen and then be given the opportunity to come to the funeral home or not, but they cannot make that decision without information. If children decide to come, they should be prepared further. They should be told the color of the rugs and walls, whether there are plants or paintings, whether there are flowers, what color the casket is, what color clothing the deceased is wearing, and that the deceased is lying down and not moving. The children should be informed so completely that when they walk into the funeral home it is almost as if they have been there before. Does it work? Children have walked into my funeral home and checked off exactly the points that I covered with their parents three hours before — ''Oh, there's a green rug, there's the painting on the wall, there are the flowers.'' When this happens, I know that the parents have used the information I have provided, and I know that the children are comfortable because the place is not strange to them. All of this draws a child into the family support network on the same side of the wall, rather than putting the child alone on the other side of the wall.

We cannot assume that parents speak to their children about death or that they know how to do so. We cannot assume that if a death occurs suddenly in the middle of the night the parents will be prepared to talk to their children about it at seven o'clock in the morning when they get up. We cannot assume that "user-friendly" information is available, that if parents were given a booklet it would apply, or even that they would read it. I used to think that talking to children about death was only the concern of parents, but another funeral director who is using my program told me that a senior citizen came to him and said, "I'm here because I want to make sure that when I die my children will provide my grandchildren with this type of information."

We cannot assume that children are not talking or thinking about a death, that they are not affected when a family pet dies or by the deaths they see every day on television, or by the death of a neighbor or classmate. We cannot assume that children are prepared in any way to come to a funeral. We cannot assume that their parents have answered their questions or that the children have asked questions. For example, I have found that about 85 percent of the children between the ages of four and twelve who come to a funeral home and see a half-closed casket do not realize or believe that the deceased's legs are in the bottom of the casket. How do I know? Because I have said to parents, address that issue with children: Walk into the funeral home and up to the casket, and say, "You know, some kids think that the whole person isn't there, so if you want us to, we'll show you the rest of the person." Some parents respond by saying "No, I don't want to do that, I don't want to deal with that." But I have found that their children will accept my invitation to have the bottom part of the casket opened so that they can look inside. I have been putting a family into a limousine and heard a child ask, "Why did they cut Grandma up?" and heard the mother say, "What do you mean they cut Grandma up?" So I have said, "She only saw half of Grandma; let's go back inside." We have gone back in, opened the bottom of the casket, and the child has said, "Oh, yes, she is all there."

Children constantly ask for this type of information. A mother said to me, "Why does my child ask if that's a dummy inside the casket? And why does she ask me how they got the dummy to look so much like Grandpa?" And I say, "What did you say to your child?" And she says that she told the child that her grandfather had died and gone to heaven. So I say, "If Grandpa died and went to heaven, who's inside the casket?"

A psychiatrist told me that he had one patient, a five-year-old boy who had been very close to his grandmother. When she died, the boy was told that Grandma had gone right up to heaven. His mother later found the boy standing on the windowsill of the apartment, about to jump out. After the boy was safely on the floor again, his mother asked him why he had been going to jump and what he thought would happen if he did. The boy said, "I would go up, just like Grandma."

So many of the points that seem like separate, discrete bits of information are actually the building materials to be fitted into a family blueprint. When I present this information to parents, they ask, "How do you expect us to put all of this together in our grief? How do you expect us to do that?" I say, "I don't expect you to do that; I expect your funeral director to do it."

Parental Grief
Over the Death of a Child

Barbara B. Johansen

This paper is my personal statement, put together from the devastating experience of my son's death, caused by cancer six years ago, when he was fourteen. He fought valiantly and suffered with the illness for almost two years. Since the time of his diagnosis, I have worked with families in the Candlelighters groups of Fairfield County, Connecticut, and Westchester County, New York, and as a telephone communication connection for parents throughout the country who contact the Center for Attitudinal Healing in Tiburon, California. In particular, I am a resource parent for the bereaved parents in Candlelighters.

I will not attempt to cover the parents' grief response to sudden death, whether caused by illness or accident. I am concerned with the grief of the parent who has experienced the death of a child through catastrophic illness.

I begin with a few quotes from a letter I received from a mother whose child had recently died. Her words are typical of the thoughts of most parents at this time:

> I would never have imagined in my worst nightmares that it was possible to miss someone as much as I miss him. My longing for him is intolerable at times — it's going to get much much worse before it gets any better. I suppose the longing will remain forever. What might get better is the ability to handle it — it's going to take a long, long time. How will we ever get through this long, cold winter? With love, career, and the comfort of our friends.

Barbara B. Johansen is Family Education Specialist and President, Change of Pace Experiences, Inc., New Canaan, CT.

© 1988 by The Haworth Press, Inc. All rights reserved.

A child's dying is one of the most devastating experiences a parent can have. It is said that when you lose a parent, you lose your past, but that when you lose your child, you lose your future.

Bereavement begins after the stages of death have been completed. Culturally, we have poor training in how to comfort the bereaved. It is extremely helpful to have a public ceremony or service to acknowledge the child's death. When a service is not held, the parents deny a social opportunity to cope with the loss.

Often it is three months before a parent is able to acknowledge the death of the child. In fact, it is not uncommon for parents to put off choosing and ordering a marker or tombstone; this allows the denial stage to continue. Often, the child's death leaves parents with inconsolable grief, ruptured lives, and personal and social adjustments that are painful and difficult. Parents show a strong tendency toward psychosocial withdrawal.

COUPLES MOURN AS INDIVIDUALS

Although the couple are parents of the same child, they do not necessarily come together at connected points during their mourning. Seldom can they lean on each other in this dramatic loss. Although they are in the same situation and have similar needs, they experience the loss from somewhat different perspectives.

It is helpful to consider the couple's past coping mechanisms. This is a new crisis, but the fight-or-flight responses are once again present, and they are likely to turn again to what they used in past times of crisis. Successfully working it out together usually requires the support of significant others. Each parent can be helped by looking at family roots—at the responses to death by his or her parents, grandparents, and significant others—in relation to how the parent is responding. Is the parent comfortable with his or her response, and if not, what changes can realistically be effected?

MOURNING PROCESS

It is helpful for parents to look at their mourning as a process time, during which they can learn much about themselves and their personal strengths and weaknesses and come to accept that life will go on. One way to do this is to look at their own and other families' previous experience with loss: where are they now in relation to the time of the child's death? What has transpired?

During the initial periods of disorientation and depression, some parents seek escape from their grief in alcohol, which can increase depression, anxiety, sleeplessness, digestive disorders, and problems with concentration. Some other parents request drugs to help them through their grief, to enable them to "carry on," or to "stop the pain." There is growing concern among medical professionals about prescribing drugs for those in mourning. The sorrow is not worked through by this type of "medical intervention" but instead is masked by the drug. Doctors are now recognizing that the most effective cure is reorientation and allowing the natural process to occur. Chemical intervention can result in chronic disorientation.

In our society, covering painful feelings is regarded as a sign of strength. It is important for parents to share their feelings and experiences with someone. Bottled-up feelings often lead to physical symptoms or behavioral changes — for example, extreme irritability or bossiness, a demanding attitude, or nervousness. It is important to keep the lines of communication open. Also, sharing activities as a family to reinforce closeness during the time of stress helps build awareness and appreciation for the new family dynamics and roles.

Spouses often do not perceive each other's expressions of pain as such. For example, the husband may stay away and work late; the wife may then think that since her husband will not talk or listen or be home with her, he does not love her or the dead child. In such situations, unnecessary misunderstandings occur, expectations go unmet, and needs are unfulfilled.

Sharing the pain with someone is important to recovery and a growing relationship, and so is time alone. Talking about the dead child is necessary and therapeutic, but it is not easy. Mention a parent who died and nobody squirms, but bring up a dead child's name and others are uncomfortable. It is easy for parents to get the feeling that they are infringing on other people's lives with their grief.

According to Davidson (1979), the mourning process includes two periods. The first of these is the disorientation period, which includes feelings of numbness, emptiness, sadness, depression, guilt, and despair, as well as emotional outbursts, weight loss or gain, anger, impaired judgment, and disorganization. The second phase of the mourning process is the reorganization period, which involves the return of feelings of hope. Learning to deal with hostile feelings is often the bridge between the two periods. Knowing and understanding this process may prove vital to parents' well-being.

Disorientation

It is useful to elaborate on some of the feelings experienced during the initial period of mourning, or disorientation:

- Numbness, felt during the initial stage of grief, is a shield against unbelievable shock—it is a stalling device that affords parents the time to muster their resources to face the loss.
- Parents often express feelings of detachment from what is happening. They say that in the midst of the funeral service they feel as if they are enclosed in a plastic bubble, judging, going through the motions, and watching from a distance.
- Shock and denial are means by which parents avoid facing the pain of separation. They claim that they "see" the dead child and have no need to grieve. "If I isolate myself from those who are talking about this, it won't have happened." Some parents immerse themselves in work or a kind of hyperactivity.
- Guilt can relate to three areas. The first of these is the health care decision—the "if" or second-guess treatment syndrome: "If the illness had been discovered sooner," or "if another treatment protocol had been chosen." There is also time-and-relationship guilt, which focuses on what the parent did not do for the child. For example, "I did not give the child enough time," and so on. For some parents, guilt also comes from the belief that the child's death is a punishment for their past. It is imperative to sort out various guilt feelings and their irrational aspects. Bereaved parents should endeavor to identify the causes of their guilt feelings and learn to forgive themselves.
- Anger is a frequent reaction against the confusion and anxiety that parents feel in connection with the death. They may feel anger toward the child, physicians and other health care pro-

fessionals, their spouse, themselves, other children, friends who have normal healthy children, and even toward God. This last can cause them to question their religious beliefs, and this, in turn, can cause guilt and anxiety. For the sake of their future inner peace, this must be explored. Anger is also an influence at a more mundane level. Day-to-day annoyances are often put aside during the child's illness, when the little things of daily life really do not matter, but then, after the child's death, "Mount Vesuvius" erupts over little things. As parents move on after the child's death, it is the little things that they are now living with and acknowledge. Conscious of these petty annoyances, it is important, if they are to remain together, that they be patient, loving, and kind, and that they lower their expectations.

The feelings of numbness, guilt, anger, and so on are expressed in many ways: crying, weeping, talking incessantly. Emotional release is vital and should be encouraged. It is important to deal with an emotion when it is first experienced. Burying it usually creates problems later. Counselors, neutral parties, and self-help groups are especially helpful in this area of coping and adjusting.

Just getting out of bed and living life as usual often seems impossible. Suicide is a common consideration, and parents have commented, "Life goes on around you while you feel incapable of going on with life" and "You wish you were dead."

For a long time, parents may be preoccupied by thoughts of the child. Everything reminds the parents of the child. Some parents are haunted by the memory of the child as he or she appeared at death or during illness. They hear the child cry or they wake up during the night to give the child medicine. They see the child in a crowd, feel the child's presence in a room, or, when they see another child of the same age, want to touch the child and, at the same time, want to run away to avoid being near.

Eventually, intense feelings of emptiness and loneliness occur, accompanied by a deep aching and a desire to hold and touch the child again. The parent feels dead inside, as if part of him or her had died with the child. All of these feelings are normal unless exaggerated or extended for a prolonged time.

Depression, which is real for almost all parents, can be continuous after the death ordeal or can come in waves. It is a painful state of unhappiness and sadness that revolves around trying to come to grips with inner feelings. Depression is experienced in a variety of ways, including preoccupation with sad thoughts, feeling tired and listless, and feeling devalued and worthless. It can affect both parents or only one, and usually has to do with a child-focused relationship.

Physical symptoms of discomfort often occur during depression. Chest pain is common, as is throat pain — possibly a defense against talking about feelings. These pains, which can occur anywhere in the body or throughout it, are usually related to an inability to share with and feel comforted by supportive people. Depression makes it difficult to concentrate on tasks, and parents easily become confused. They have difficulty keeping up at work, and let others' needs go unmet. They may have difficulty making decisions or, conversely, may make decisions impulsively without weighing their long-term effects. Depression is a form of anger turned back on the self that can be extremely self-destructive.

Complicating these feelings is the fact that at this time the parents must make two major decisions. The first is what they should do with the child's clothing, furniture, and toys? The parents often have differing opinions. It is certainly important that the child's room not become a museum, but time should be made for open discussion. The second momentous decision is whether or not they should have another child. Not immediately, the "experts" recommend. No child can ever be a replacement; hence, it is wise for parents to wait a reasonable length of time to share and work through their grief before building a new family structure.

Reorganization

After parents have accepted a child's death intellectually, they still experience painful psychological and physical feelings. It may take some parents several years to achieve resolution, recovery, and reorganization. For parents, the first steps toward working through these "three Rs" are knowing that their reactions are not abnormal, learning to deal with their feelings, and knowing that others have found their way out of this dark tunnel. "Recovery" is often determined by how parents react following the death and how they are treated by others during the early, most profound stage of grief. The parents who move through the grief process most quickly are those who stop asking "Why?" (there is no acceptable answer); who accept the truth of the child's death; who include the death as part of life; who do not let their lives revolve around the child's death; and who afford patience to themselves and their spouses.

Gradually, the painful times become shorter and less frequent, a "hardship" that parents learn to live with. They will always remember the child, and they become capable of recalling some of the good moments. They become involved again with life activities and see options and possibilities for the future. The pain of loss becomes less intense, good days outbalance the bad, and the parents are able to take pleasure without guilt, to laugh again, and finally to talk about happy memories of their child without being overwhelmed by grief. Thus, tragic loss can give rise to renewed meaning and personal growth.

It is helpful if the parents are aware of the process they are going through and if they are able to emphasize patience with self and love of self and spouse even amid the confusion. Staying in the present — not looking back or planning the future — is extremely helpful. Life will go on, although it will be difficult. The idea is to try to avoid a "pity party" by learning to live in the present and being fully alive. It is important to step away from mourning when it is over.

HISTORY AND THE ROAD TO RECOVERY

At the turn of the century, losing a child was a common experience. There were role models to follow. Parents had others close to them who had shared the same experience. Today, more than 94,000 children under the age of twenty-four die annually (National Center for Health Statistics 1987), but most parents grapple with their grief alone. Many couples suffer marital disturbances following the death of a child, the usual source being lack of understanding of each other. Indeed, Kubler-Ross (1973) noted that in her experience approximately seventy percent of bereaved couples experience serious marital problems within the first year after a child's death. Blame can be devastating in this regard. A parent who has an inclination toward blame of either self or spouse should be urged to seek psychiatric help. Preventive medicine in this situation comprises counseling and self-help groups. Each parent can do much to clarify misunderstandings and avert marital discord.

Neighbors and others are often too embarrassed to be of much comfort. Consequently, parents tend to isolate themselves and others tend to stay away because they too are feeling deep grief over the child's death. Others feel helpless and therefore often do nothing.

In 1969, Father Simon Stephens, an Anglican priest in Coventry, England, founded Compassionate Friends, an organization through which bereaved parents provide each other with mutual support. The impetus for establishing the organization grew out of his experience in bringing together two couples whose children had died on the same day and the realization that sharing grief can bring healing and wholeness (Stephens 1973). Today there are chapters of Compassionate Friends throughout the United States. In addition, medical centers and community organizations, realizing the positive effects of self-help programs, are forming groups to help the bereaved.

Jane Brody (1983), columnist and writer, has discussed two main resources, friends and relatives, and specified the ways they can help bereaved parents:

- Let caring show—reach out even if you feel helpless.
- Make yourself available to listen, run errands, and help with other children, etc.
- Say you're sorry about what happened—don't suggest they should be grateful for other children or they can have another child—no child can be replaced.
- Let them fully express their grief—don't suggest they should be feeling better by now.
- Encourage them to be patient and not expect too much of themselves.
- Allow them to talk about qualities of the child.
- Don't try to find something positive about the child's death.

- Reassure them that they did everything they could to help the child. Don't criticize the medical care the child received.
- Pay special attention to surviving siblings, who often are neglected in time of intense parental grief.

Support groups offer parents the hope that they will be able to go on, reprieve from a strained, lonely existence, a chance to sort through what has happened, an opportunity to find role models for how to cope, and the ability to talk about the child and their experiences in an accepting and supportive atmosphere. Support groups also offer guides to explain some of the basic, universal reactions. Someone who has been there before can help others; the group can act as a defusing agent for the parents. The time discrepancy between public expectations and the reality of recovery—often an explosive issue—can be explored. In self-help groups, parents are sometimes the ones who are supported and sometimes the ones who give support. This shared experience can be an opportunity for growth.

Following a child's death, parents often assure each other that their feelings are "normal," that they are not going crazy, and, if the child experienced a prolonged illness, that they are feeling relief at the child's death, knowing that the child will no longer be suffering. Inwardly, they nevertheless question themselves. In the group setting, through the sharing of conversation, books, films, and professional presentations, they gain new insights and understandings about particular problems and situations. Sometimes they need more help in dealing with their feelings—other parents can encourage those who need extra professional counseling but are reluctant to seek it.

Building on support systems that were present during the child's illness requires the least amount of effort to produce the positive support needed during bereavement. The Candlelighters and community groups can provide this support. I believe that it is important for medical centers to acknowledge this fact and to offer continuing support systems during bereavement. Unless they extend a support network for a reasonable time, the institutions are buying into the "instant cure culture" and ignoring a social and moral obligation to families.

Despite the help and support of family, friends, self-help groups, and professionals, there inevitably are "special" days when sadness is intense. Holidays are an obvious example. Although there is no way of getting around them, it seems to help parents, again, if they can focus on the present rather than on the past or the future and remembering that they have an obligation to the remaining family and to themselves to reach out for whatever joy or pleasure such bittersweet occasions may bring. Bereaved parents should also be encouraged to plan a change of scene, a break in tradition, or the addition of some new faces at holiday times. It is normal for periods of sadness to recur for many years, particularly on special dates, but present occasions should not be blurred by yearning toward the past.

According to behavioral researchers, loving and caring for a pet can help those who are bereaved. Pets are uncritical, consistently loving, and do not give orders. Pets offer a dependable welcome and a feeling of security. Through talking about their pets, uncommunicative individuals can become more socially active. Studies indicate that touching animals is a source of comfort that might not be available or even desirable from other people. Parents who have had to care for a dying child over a long period may respond well to caring for a friendly new pet.

Research indicates that parents who have faith in God seem to be helped considerably by this belief. For parents without this faith, death seems to affect them as an even greater tragedy. Many parents question God and their belief systems after the death of their child. Because belief systems are highly personal, as are individuals' responses to a child's death, they can be another stumbling block for the couple to struggle with. Accepting each other's beliefs in relation to the death of their child, although profoundly difficult, can bring growth on many levels.

Pinkson (1985) has discussed the positive effects that a child's death at home can have on all concerned. Appropriate farewells can be made in a "natural" way in a comfortable setting. It is extremely helpful for the parents as well as siblings to share these last moments in their own familiar, supportive atmosphere, where grief can be openly and honestly shared.

Kubler-Ross has often noted that confronting and accepting the inevitability of one's own death can help one to attain inner peace. Parents must be encouraged to continue living, using each moment as best they can. Accepting the confusion of self and spouse with love and patience can be the beginning of recovery.

REFERENCES

Brody, J. 1983. "People Who Are Depressed by the Loss of a Relative or Friend Can Learn to Love and Care for a Pet." *The New York Times*, Wed., Feb. 16, Section C, p. 15.

Davidson, G. 1979. *Death of the Wished-For Child* (videotape). Clobber Film Laboratories, Chicago, IL.

National Center for Health Statistics. 1971. "Monthly Statistics Report" 36(5), Aug. 26th. U.S. Department of Health and Human Services.

Kubler-Ross, E. 1973. In foreword to S. Stevens, *Death Comes Home*. New York: Morehouse Barlow.

Pinkson, T. *Do They Celebrate Christmas in Heaven?* Farmingdale, NY: Coleman Publishing.

D